New Faces

CAUTION:
USE WITH DEVOTION

Some beauty books tell you what to put on your face, and others what to eat for it, and still others how to behave to be beautiful. Some—often expensive—show you magic exercises to smooth away wrinkles and lines. But *this* little beauty book includes them all— cosmetics, diet, exercises and even the art of serenity. NEW FACES can be as valuable to you as your favorite jewel if you use it with the same devotion.

BOOKS BY LINDA CLARK

Be Slim and Healthy
Light on Your Health Problems
Help Yourself to Health
Secrets of Health and Beauty
Stay Young Longer
Get Well Naturally
Know Your Nutrition

Completely Illustrated

New Faces

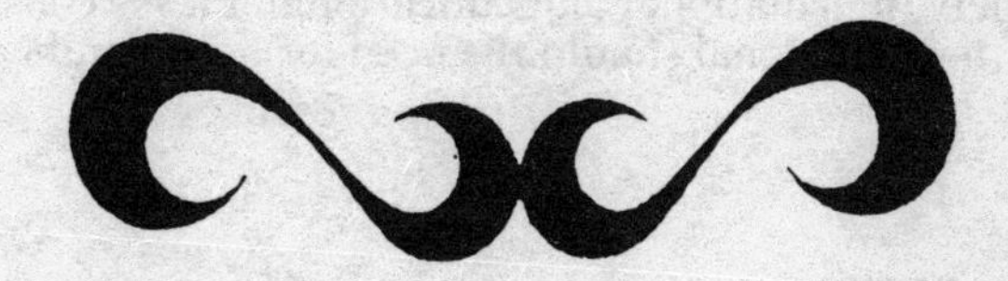

LINDA CLARK

Illustrations by Charles Mazoujian

Foreword by Barbara Hegne
author of *Everywoman's Every Day Exercise and Nutrition Plan*

Keats Publishing, Inc. New Canaan, Connecticut

New Faces is not intended as medical advice. Its intent is solely informational and educational. Please consult a health professional should the need for one be indicated.

NEW FACES
Originally published as *Face Improvement Through Exercise and Nutrition.*

Printed in the United States of America

Library of Congress Catalog Card Number: 72-97919

ISBN: 0-87983-515-X

Published by Keats Publishing, Inc.
27 Pine Street (Box 876)
New Canaan, Connecticut 06840

Dedicated
to all women who care enough
to look their best

Contents

Foreword

"Mirror, mirror on the wall, who is fairest of all?" The mirror reflected Snow White's face as pleasant, beautiful and fair to gaze upon; her beauty emerged from the inside, fresh, healthy, and clean. The wicked queen's face was sealed in a permanent frown as she spent her time scowling and constantly wrinkling her face in discontent.

If the wicked queen could read Linda Clark's *New Faces*, she would learn that wrinkles are only skin deep and with the perfect "smile-up" exercise, a change of attitude and a few healthful habits, she could be in fair competition with Snow White.

The world is moving at such a rapid pace that people have little time for storybooks, and less time for exercise. When they do manage an hour at the spa, their time is spent frantically attacking the fat on the hips, thighs and buttocks, and little or no thought is given the face.

In my twenty years of teaching health, nutrition and fitness, I have read thousands of books and articles on those subjects, many of which have very detailed programs. Too often the routines are complicated and time-consuming; and people become discouraged and abandon the effort. *New Faces* has solved the problem of the "I don't have time and it's too hard" syndrome.

Many times we forget that the face is an

extension of our body, and our addictions and food habits show through for all the world to see. Linda Clark makes us aware of how our lifestyle affects health and beauty. She points out some of the culprits that rob us of our beauty: alcohol, drugs, cigarette smoking, weather, dramatic weight loss, lack of sleep, poor dieting and sunbathing. Ms. Clark shows us how to combat the beauty enemies through nutritional diet, organic facial products, positive attitude, and specific exercises that tighten and strengthen the underlying facial muscles. She reveals tips and tricks that national makeup artists, models and movie stars use to keep their perfect beauty image before the camera, and addresses some commonly asked questions regarding face-exercise machines, massage, and cosmetic surgery (face lifts).

For most women, keeping the face in good shape means a drawer full of every imaginable cosmetic. Ms. Clark suggests natural food cosmetics without sprays or additives. We learn that the skin is a living, breathing, absorbing organ, and that what goes on the face should have top priority.

I fell into the cosmetic chemical trap when I was in my early twenties. I began having daily headaches of which I attributed to allergies—then, after a lot of expensive and tiresome tests, I found I was sensitive to the chemicals in my lipstick, and was creating my own problems.

I learned much from *New Faces*, and I am now using the "smile-up" exercise in my own classes. It is simple and effective. It works about 100 muscles of the face, and because of the effects of the smile itself, my students leave class feeling like a million dollars. I have to admit that unless you are in a class with other people doing facial exercises, you may feel odd making an "O" with your mouth, sticking your tongue out or sucking your cheeks inward, but *New Faces* gives you the uncomplicated directions for doing it in the privacy of your home.

Linda Clark is looked upon as one of the leading authorities in the field of health and nutrition and she applies that knowledge to this book. She is a dynamic writer who gets the point across honestly without making you feel you are getting a beating for not being perfect. She is helpful in informing readers of the options and the consequences, and leaving the choice up to them. Through it all, the reader gets the feeling they are being gently directed toward a goal that will be of benefit to them.

Linda Clark was best known as a nutritional reporter, but her expertise went beyond that. In *New Faces* she has called upon well-known physicians and beauty advisors to present a total beauty and health picture. I feel confident when I read any of her works that she has already attended to the difficult task of proving out what she presents. My respect for her is based on her accurate knowledge and her record of in-depth research.

I am honored to be asked to write the foreword to a book by someone I have looked up to for many years. I have used Linda Clark's suggestions, information and advice in my professional work and in my personal life.

So, with Linda Clark as your guide, you have

your opportunity to renew and revitalize your self and your appearance. Open the book and . . . face up to it.

BARBARA HEGNE
May 1990

1

ABOUT YOUR FACE

Chapter One

Your Face Is Your Billboard

You have heard the expression, "Your face is your fortune." For models, entertainers and politicians, this may be true. It may or may not apply to others. There is one thing, however, that applies to everyone. Your face is your billboard! Your face reveals to others whether you are pleasant or unpleasant; happy or sad; approachable, contented, sympathetic, friendly, or the reverse. In short, your face is perhaps the most important part of your image. When a person meets you, the first thing he looks at is your face. He takes a general sounding of you via your hair, your body, your dress, your grooming and your voice. But your face serves as a map that he searches intently, perhaps unconsciously, for clues on how to proceed in his communication with you.

Everything you are can be read in your face. It is your major link with humanity.

Your face can also tell doctors and nutritionists about your health. It often gives them clues to the diagnoses of some diseases as well as their treatment. For centuries the American Indians considered the face a health map of the entire body. Lines and other signs of the face enabled them to diagnose body ailments and suggest remedies.

This is not so farfetched as it sounds. Today, there is a comparatively new method of physical diagnosis and treatment called *Contact Therapy*. This method is somewhat similar to *Acupuncture*, which divides the body into invisible parallel zones running vertically from head to foot. Acupuncture points located anywhere in these zones are said to influence different parts of the body. Treatment at the correct points is said to bring improvement to the specific area needing help. Acupuncture, of course, is done by inserting fine needles into certain points in the body zones. It has been used successfully by the Chinese for many generations.

Zone therapy, or *Reflexology*, as it is sometimes called, deals with the apparent endings of these same zones on the bottom of the feet. A map of the feet indicates to reflexologists which areas of the body each nerve ending influences. Many patients and therapists report definite improvement by treatment on these specific foot points, not by inserting a needle, but by pressing and massaging any foot area that is sensitive or painful. This, in turn, relieves congestion or constriction there as well as elsewhere in the body. This may explain why, if your feet hurt, you hurt all over.

The newer zonal method, Contact Therapy, deals with the zone endings at the other end of the body: the head and face. There is at least one book on this subject, with a map of the face and head showing the specific points that are related to various body areas, glands and organs. The principle of Contact Therapy is that if there is tenderness or soreness at any of the facial (or head) points, there is congestion in the corresponding part of the body. Treatment is simple. It requires only firm pressure, not massage, by the finger tips on these points. Probing with your fingers you can locate these face or head areas yourself, by trial and error. If you find a sore place, whether or not you know which body area it affects, the theory is that if you will press firmly, no matter how painful the spot, for a few minutes each day, the soreness will eventually subside. According to Contact Therapy, the corresponding body disturbance will also be improved. There are many dramatic reports of health improvement by this method.

I have described these pressure points and their locations, because your face *is* connected with the rest of your body and registers what is going on there. Your face, as well as your feet, reflects what is happening. Watch any woman shopper who has been on her feet for hours in tight-fitting, uncomfortable, or too high-heeled shoes. The agony she is feeling in her feet is registered in her face. Conversely, one woman who began to do face exercises, told me she felt better all over, an unexpected and subtle dividend derived from face exercises.

Thus, your face can report the physical condition of your body as well as mirror your emotions. Your eyes are a part of your face, too. Eyes can express love, interest in others, joy, happiness and good humor, or hate and resentment. Or they can appear dull and vacant-looking, as they often are in those who are drug addicts.

Your face deserves all the help it can get. Let's see what to do about it.

2

DIET AND YOUR FACE

Chapter Two

The Right Kind of Diet For Your Face

Your face tells nutritionists and doctors what you are or are not eating. The clues are easy to see for those who know what to look for.

The Effect of Oils

If your skin is dry and flaky and becomes lined easily, it is a clue that you are deficient in oils. Those who shudder at eating vegetable oils for fear of gaining weight have a surprise in store. Researchers find that eating fat helps to burn up excess body fat. Many who have tried every way to lose weight and failed have succeeded by adding several tablespoons of natural vegetable oil to their diet daily. Oils also give your skin a sheen and create a plumper, younger look, as compared to the wizened prune-face so common in older people. Oils can be added to salads, or poured into the blender with fruit or vegetable drinks and whizzed thoroughly. (You will never know they are there.)

I have seen dry skin (and hair) develop a sheen within two short weeks after cod liver oil was included in the diet. If you think "Ugh" about cod liver oil, I don't blame you. But if you use one tablespoon of refrigerated *mint-flavored* cod liver oil, combined with two tablespoons of cold orange juice, both shaken well in a small jar reserved for this purpose (to keep the flavor and odor from other containers), you will be surprised at how palatable it is. Taken at bedtime, it is well-assimilated and tasty, I assure you. As a former cod liver oil hater, I was converted to it used in this way. I have, in turn, converted others, providing it *is* used in this way.

Various eczemas as well as falling hair have been noted in animals deficient in oils. So if you wish a dewy skin, add several tablespoons of various vegetable oils in one form or another to your daily diet.

The Role of Protein

Another thing your face tells about your diet is whether or not you are getting enough protein. The body, including the skin, is made mostly of protein; and protein *must* be used daily by the body to replace that lost in a myriad of needs by organs, glands and other body functions. If you suffer from a protein deficiency, your skin is going to show the lack by becoming slack and loose, and the protein-deprived muscles that hold up your face are going to weaken and droop. A skin deficient in protein becomes wrinkled early and develops folds. Lecithin added to the diet as well as to cosmetics encourages skin plumping (Lecithin is found in health stores.)

Athletes are fed protein to strengthen their body muscles. Carbohydrates make for flabby muscles (and skin). Thus, protein—or its lack—affects the face as well as the body. For a firm body and an unlined skin, look to your protein intake.

Weather

Weather, too, can play havoc with your face. Those who are sun worshippers, and stubbornly expose themselves to the sun for hours, may look temporarily healthy, but they are also the ones who age earliest. They develop the weather-beaten faces found in sailors and desert natives who have been exposed to the relentless sun. Women with the peaches-and-cream complexions that last well into old age are those who live in a moist climate, as in England. They wear wide-brimmed hats or protect their skins from the sun with parasols as many Oriental women do. Our Victorian predecessors had beautiful, fair, fine-textured skin. They would not be seen without a large hat and often a parasol as well. This custom is now returning because women have found that sun worshipping makes them look far older, often irreversibly, than those who have protected their skins from all but a *small amount* of morning or afternoon sun, never the midday burning rays. Skin cancer is, of course, another well-known result of too much sunning.

So it pays to wear a hat when exposed to the sun. One woman, a famous hostess who lives near me, keeps a collection of large hats available for her guests who wish to enjoy the California sun on her patio or the beach. She is actually protecting the beauty of their faces. Sun and wind dry up moisture in the face, and a lack of moisture can create wrinkles in no time. Compare the skin of women who live in humid versus dry climates!

Raw Food

A muddy skin is unattractive, too. It is usually due to lack of fresh, raw food. Raw food, whether vegetables used in salads or fresh fruit used as desserts or snacks, contains enzymes that are the body's housecleaners and keep the bloodstream cleaner. Fresh raw food results in brighter, clearer eyes, an important factor in a beautiful face, as well as a fresh, clear complexion. Movie and television stars have learned this secret and eat generously of raw foods, both vegetables and fruits.

No-No's

Stars in the entertainment field have also learned another lesson about what *not* to put into their bodies: alcohol and tobacco. Those who have learned the hard way state that if they wish to appear fresh, and looking their best before the camera or public, they dare not drink alcohol (a three-ounce glass of dry wine with dinner can be the only exception).

A recent Blue Cross report states that smoking has definitely been found to cause wrinkles.

Drugs do not encourage good skin. They also can encourage that "dead" expression in the eyes.

Natural Foods and Supplements

Natural, organic wholesome food, without sprays or additives, can contribute to a clear skin. And since so much food these days is deficient in the vitamins and minerals eaten by our grandparents, supplemental vitamins and minerals, especially the latter, are a *must* to make up for this deficiency in our food. Actually, supplemental minerals are becoming more important than vitamins, because, without them, vitamins cannot deliver their punch. Natural vitamin and mineral supplements derived from food are more complete than individual chemical substances which have been synthesized. If you have not already investigated your health store, now is the time. Not only are natural foods and supplements available there, but natural cosmetics as well.

Natural Cosmetics

Cosmetics made from natural food sources, not chemicals, should be included in the diet for your face. Unlike the food you eat, these natural substances are put *on* the skin (which scientists now know can be fed), instead of into the body via the mouth. Either way, they work to improve your face. I have told how you can find, or make at home, natural cosmetics in my book, *Secrets of Health and Beauty.** You will find the whole fascinating story told there.

Recent information has shown that the application of creams and oils helps the face. But creams and oils are not the whole story; moisture is important, too. A researcher learned this when he applied oils to dried leather without good results. But when he submerged the same leather in water, the wrinkles smoothed out and the skin plumped up. It was this finding that led to the discovery of moisturizers in cosmetics. They are not the only substances needed, however, for a good diet for the face. Proteins, minerals, and vitamins are needed, too, for application to the skin.

The face, as well as the body, needs to be given the right things to eat and drink. And, as Aida Grey, the Hollywood makeup expert says, the diet for the face needs to be as varied as the diet for the body. Rather than eating the same old things every day, one nutritionist suggests that you should eat a different menu every day in the month to assure your body getting everything it needs. Your skin benefits from a change in cosmetics too, though perhaps not daily, so that it, too, can enjoy a full supply of nature's bounty.

Other things are necessary to insure good looks. Let us see in the next chapter what they are.

---

*Linda Clark, *Secrets of Health and Beauty*, Pyramid.

3

HELP FOR YOUR FACE

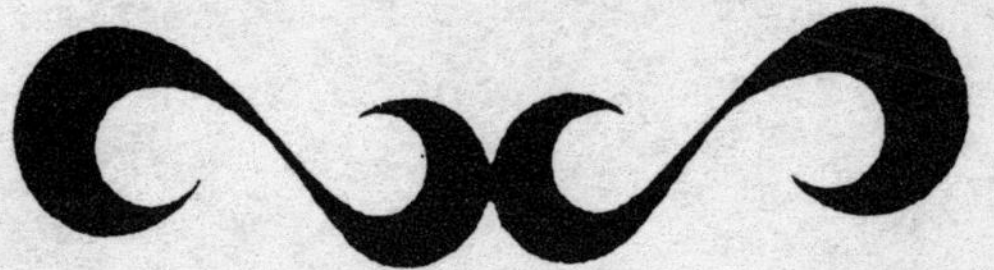

Chapter Three

Basic Ways to Help Your Face

You can eat the best diet in the world, but if you do not have good circulation to deliver the goodies to various parts of the body, that good diet may be less effective than it should be. People who want firm, lithe bodies, find that body exercise helps in two ways: one, by increasing the circulation of fresh blood, containing the nutrients derived from the diet, to all areas of the body, including the face; two, by strengthening the muscles. Exercise shortens loose, slack muscles and makes them firm and taut. It also helps to diminish the fat around those muscles. In an animal, the muscles exercised the most are surrounded by the least amount of fatty tissue. Exercised dogs or horses are firm and lithe, whereas unexercised, lazy animals are fat and flabby. Improved circulation and face exercise do exactly the same things for the face as for the body.

The face is part of the body and needs exercise, too. You may not realize it, but there are fifty-five muscles in your face. Some are overused, some underused, others incorrectly used. As people grow older, their circulation slows down. Children have nearly 100 per cent perfect circulation. Very elderly people may have only about 25 per cent, whereas middle-aged people may have a percentage anywhere in between. Poor circulation can result in undernourished as well as weakened and lengthened muscles, muscles similar to a rubber band that is permanently stretched. As muscles stretch, the face droops and sags. But these flabby muscles can be firmed and shortened by face exercises so that they can pull up and hold up the face again. If exercise can recondition the body (and we know it can), it can also help recondition the face.

Animals, which walk on all fours, do not develop drooping, sagging faces as they get older. But humans do because they stand upright. The face is the area farthest from the feet, and it is constantly pulled downward by gravity. One way to combat this gravity down-pull as well as speed up poor circulation is to lie on a slant board, with your feet about eighteen inches above your head so that the blood rushes automatically to your head and face. This position encourages the muscles to reverse their pull of gravity. If you look at your face in a mirror while you are lying in the slant position, you will see that it has become naturally lifted. One television and movie star believes that if you spend at least twenty minutes a day on a slant board, you will never need a surgical face lift. You can buy slant boards, or you can make your own. Merely prop up one end of a wide board, purchased from a lumber store, on bricks so that your feet are approximately eighteen inches higher than your head. There is nothing more refreshing than a few minutes spent in this position when you are fagged. University researchers find that it clears your thinking, and relieves the strain of gravity pull on organs throughout your entire body. It also helps your face. You look and feel better all over afterward. Elderly people, particularly those with high blood pressure, should start out with less than twenty minutes a day in a slant position and get up slowly from that position. If you have any questions, ask your doctor.

Don't confuse skin problems with muscle problems. Surface treatment of the skin does *not* help the underlying muscles, which may be the cause of your drooping face. However, exercise can help turn a flabby muscle into a firmer one, thus improving the tissues lying between the muscle and the skin, and plumping them up like a pillow. In many cases this may result in firming or tightening the skin. By this method some wrinkles may be lessened or even removed.

All wrinkles are *creases*. Many of them, such as furrows between the brows or crow's-feet beside the eyes, often develop from continuous frowning and squinting. If these bad habits are perpetuated, the creases will return as fast as you iron them out. (The wrinkle-removing methods are discussed later in this book.) Actually, squinting and frowning are undesirable forms of face exercise.

Weight loss can often add years to the face because the muscles lose protein, become weak and cannot hold up the tissues, which in turn lose their plumpness. If adequate protein is supplied during a reducing diet, and if face exercises are continued, the face should respond and quickly bounce back to normal.

Body repair is taking place constantly, provided the right repair materials are fed to the body. Repair is especially effective during sleep, when the expenditure of energy is low. Thus, too little sleep can affect your face. When you look at yourself in the mirror after too little, or a poor night's sleep, your haggard face is mute testimony to the fact.

A healthy face is an attractive face. Allover body exercise promotes better circulation, better health, improved skin color, brighter, clearer eyes. Allover exercise should be done out-of-doors if possible, to encourage deeper breathing, which helps the body to rid itself of toxins through the lungs. Look at anyone who plays golf, swims, gardens, or merely walks a lot out-of-doors. It shows in the face. This person feels better and looks more vibrant than one who remains constantly indoors. An appearance of well-being applies to one's face as well as body.

One more thing that affects your face: your thoughts. People who are grumpy, resentful, or carrying a chip on the shoulder show it in their faces. This is not good advertising. A happy, cheerful face, with smiling eyes, attracts people. An expression of hate, disgust or disinterest in others repels them. Those who are solely interested in their own problems are not as attractive as those who are interested in and sympathetic with others. People can read the news in your face and the expression of your eyes, and react to you accordingly.

Your own evaluation of yourself is also important. I have told the story in another book*

---

*Linda Clark, *Help Yourself to Health*, Pyramid.

about a waitress whom everyone avoided. She perpetually wore a sour look and everyone shunned her if possible. Finally someone asked her why she was always so disagreeable. She said, "Why shouldn't I be disagreeable? Look at me. Every morning I look at myself in the mirror and say, 'You ugly thing!' and it puts me out of sorts for the whole day."

Then someone suggested to her that, instead, she look in the mirror every day and say to herself, "I am kind, pleasant and becoming more attractive." It actually worked! She became a different person: cheerful, kind, and pleasant to others. Her facial appearance actually became more attractive. This is because the message got through to her subconscious mind and helped produce better results.

I told the story in the same book of another woman who was not only ill, but discontented with her lot. She truly had an unattractive face. She suddenly decided that she was concentrating on her own problems to the exclusion of others, and was too self-centered. She prayed to be a channel of love toward others. In due time her entire personality changed for the better, and people began to consider her beautiful. A radiance had replaced the darkness in her expression.

A pretty or handsome face should not be a goal in itself. People admire it, yes, but the face must be warmed by an inner glow. If you don't believe it, look at any mannikin in a store window. The features are perfect but leave the onlooker as cold as the lifeless expression in the mannikin's eyes.

To gain the aid of your subconscious in improving your face as well as your personality, make a strong mental movie of yourself every night on going to sleep (a good time to impress your subconscious). Visualize yourself as you want to be, instead of as you are. This, when coupled with the other self-helps in this book, will produce far better and faster results.

In summary, to repair and improve your face, it is necessary to:

—Eat the right diet
—Use the right kind of natural cosmetics
—Watch your alcohol and smoking
—Get enough sleep
—Get enough outdoor exercise
—Use a slant board to encourage circulation
—Do face exercises for circulation, firmness and muscle strength
—Watch your thinking!

4

SOME QUESTIONS AND ANSWERS

Chapter Four

Questions and Answers About Your Face

Q. What about massage? Does it help your face?
A. It can help to encourage better circulation, but indiscriminate massage by untrained operators can do more harm than good. The skin and muscles may be pulled, stretched and weakened, and, like permanently stretched rubber bands may never again return to normal. The correct type of safe face massage is explained in the chapter on wrinkles.

Q. Is a chin strap, or those gadgets that are supposed to hold up the face, helpful?
A. A chin strap, or a temporary "face-lift" gadget is similar to a girdle. It holds your muscles up temporarily, but does not strengthen them. They droop the minute the gadget is removed. On the other hand, body and face exercises, plus the correct diet, strengthen the muscles to help them stay up on their own.

Q. Do you believe a surgical face-lift is necessary?
A. This is up to the individual. It is not the final answer, since one face-lift is often followed by another. Some plastic surgeons encourage their patients to use face exercises first, to strengthen

the muscles, thus increasing the success of the surgical face-lift; or to use face exercises *instead* of the face-lift, depending on the person. There are various women noted in history who have retained their youthful appearance throughout their lives without a face-lift. But you must co-operate with nature, not defy it, if you wish to avoid the need for a face-lift. If you burn the candle at both ends—eat unwisely, take drugs, use unlimited tobacco and alcohol, eat foods empty of repair materials, get too little sleep and exercise—you could create the need for a face-lift.

Q. How long does it take to recondition a face through exercise?
A. It depends on how far gone it is! Younger people should start the minute (or before) they note the first sign of aging and keep it up the rest of their lives, just as they should do regular body exercise.

One face-exercise expert who demonstrated facial exercises on television produced some almost instantaneous results, as did watchers of the program who tried the same exercises. But regular exercise is needed to maintain this improvement. Some types of face faults need more time than others.

Q. What about face-exercise machines?
A. A machine is a lazy woman's exerciser. If the person understands the anatomy of her face and is regular with her own exercises, she will have as good or better results. Machines, which contract the underlying muscles, have been helpful

if used regularly, though they may not speed the circulation as thoroughly as self-exercising. However, though they are not dangerous, many face machines have been banned because of claims made for their use. If you have a machine, by all means use it, and for faster results supplement it with your own exercises. If you do not have one, don't fret. You can do it yourself.

5

TIPS FOR SUCCESS

Chapter Five

Tips For Success

To be successful, face exercises should be done regularly. Choose a time of day, consistently scheduled, when you can depend upon not being interrupted. Do them on a slant board. Or, close your bathroom door, sit comfortably before a mirror, and go to work. Establish the habit, just as automatically as you brush your teeth, either in the morning before you apply your make-up, or the last thing at night after you have removed it. The time of day is least important, provided you just *do* them!

You may need a little time to learn the face-exercise routine required for your particular problems. But once learned, the total exercises may take no longer than ten minutes daily. When you see decided improvement, indicating that the muscles have become stronger, you may not need to do the exercises as often; perhaps only on alternate days, then twice weekly and, finally, once a week. Face exercise will prove to be one of the best investments of time for good looks that you have ever made. Most models and film and television stars do them daily without fail.

Whenever possible, do your face exercises on a slant board. This may be the only time you do them each day or may be an extra time during the day when you are relaxing. Coaxing fresh circulation to the face, until the face feels warm, takes longer in an upright position. Doing them while lying on a slant board encourages this warmth more quickly and hastens the results by speeding the circulation to the face. This is because gravity is reversed during the slant position and circulation is automatically increased.

Dr. Rudolf Drobil, of Vienna, believes that face exercises are useless unless performed against resistance. This theory will be explained in later chapters.

Before choosing your exercises, analyze your special problems and select the exercises to treat them. But regardless of the exercises you choose, always start with, and end with, the smile-up exercise. This one helps to shorten or tighten the muscles that pull up the entire face as well as to tighten the under-chin area. If you have a few spare seconds during the day—as you are waiting at a traffic light, for the water to boil, or the phone to ring—do the smile-up exercise a few times. Good results will be faster.

6

ABOUT WRINKLES

Chapter Six

Wrinkles

When you choose, learn and start to use the face exercises you need for your particular problems, you can expect some lessening of wrinkles as a result of the exercises themselves. It is true that wrinkles are only skin-deep, but, as stated previously, face exercises plump up the underlying tissues, which lie between the muscles and the skin, giving the skin more support. This added support can help tighten and smooth the skin just as plumping up the filling in a pillow tightens and smooths the pillow cover. But other measures are also needed to help iron out wrinkles.

If the body is undernourished, particularly in proteins and oils, the facial tissues cannot properly develop good tone in the first place! The face is just an extension of the body and has the same needs, plus extra need for circulation and moisture. Cosmetics containing protein, oils and moisture, accompanied by good circulation, can help prevent or repair facial lines. Certain types of massage, if the rules are followed *exactly*, also help smooth out wrinkles, too.

There will be much faster success with wrinkle removal if bad habits (often done unconsciously) of grimacing, squinting, frowning, and continuously raising and wrinkling the forehead while talking, are discontinued. Even though the creases which result may be largely smoothed away, if your habits persist, you will continue to deepen the wrinkles as fast as you try to erase them. By regularly employing the following massage methods, and maintaining a serene expression as much as possible, you should be able to reduce wrinkles to a minimum.

The under-eye area is the average woman's greatest complaint. Lines develop here more rapidly than elsewhere on the face. This is because the under-eye area has a thinner underlying cushion of fatty cells and fewer sebaceous glands. The skin in this area is extremely fragile, and any harsh rubbing, probing, stretching or pulling can produce more lines, as well as loose skin that may never recover. If, however, you observe the following rules, you have nothing to fear and improvement is definitely possible.

Don Nelson, a cosmetologist and makeup artist for television and photography, cautions women not to use even the index finger in applying face creams.* He says, "The touch of this finger becomes too forceful and can damage delicate muscle fibers. Instead, use the ball of the second and third fingers, in a gentle upward and outward movement, to roll on cleansers, creams and makeup." He believes that using a light touch with the second and third fingers actually helps to firm the face.

Jessica Krane agrees.** She warns, "Each of us

**Family Circle*, May 1971.

**Jessica Krane, *How to Use Your Hands to Save Your Face*, Hawthorne Books, Inc.

is responsible for the speed of our own aging. . . . Starting in childhood, heavy-handed touching of the face and neck can prove disastrous!" She explains that the face damaged by touch and pull loses its elasticity and firmness and eventually becomes droopy and baggy. As a former pianist, she recommends, when touching the face, to use a pianissimo touch (as soft as possible). She believes in stroking very gently upward and outward, never downward. It is also wise to stroke the lined areas in the opposite direction from which the lines are developing. Some facial consultants suggest "finger printing" or tapping lightly with the balls of the fingers, for applying cosmetics to the fragile eye areas.

Any cosmetics applied to lines under the eye should be tapped in with the finger tip, not rubbed, to avoid stretching the delicate skin. On any other area, when applying oil, cream or any cosmetic, tense the area, then rub *across*, not with the wrinkle.

There is another school of thought on treatment to remove wrinkles. This treatment, which must be done with care, is just the opposite of the tender-loving-care method described above. One exponent of this school was the late Sanford Bennett. He said,* "The true secret of restoring to the skin the smoothness of youth is friction. The skin can be polished and the wrinkles rubbed out like any other piece of leather, and the palms of the hands and tips of the fingers are the very best tools to use for that purpose." The book contains two pictures of Mr.

---

*Sanford Bennett, *Old Age, Its Causes and Prevention.* (Out of print).

Bennett, known as the man who grew young at seventy. In the first, taken at age fifty, Mr. Bennett looks like the father of himself as portrayed in the second picture, at seventy-two years of age.

Sanford Bennett added, "Use a lubricant of some kind to prevent chafing. To keep the skin in place while you rub, lightly stretch the skin between the first and second fingers of one hand and rub with the fingers or palm of the other. Don't be too energetic at first."

Mr. Bennett believed that if the skin is gradually educated to accept friction, it will not be loosened. His pictures certainly provide proof that it can be done.

The late Frederick M. Rossiter, M.D., a specialist in facial anatomy, whose face was smooth and young looking at sixty-nine, suggested an even safer way to massage the face firmly, so that the skin will not be stretched or loosened. He told how he removed wrinkles in his book, *Face Culture.** He stated that merely moving the fingers back and forth on the skin can be undeniably soothing and pleasant, but is of no benefit in removing wrinkles or strengthening muscles. His method is this: if you *contract* a muscle, and hold it tense while you massage the area of skin overlying it with fingers or palms, you may improve both skin and muscles. In this way, it is safe to massage away wrinkles and encourage circulation at the same time. Your face will become pink and warm. By contracting the area, the skin is not stretched or loosened, Dr. Rossiter has assured us.

*Frederick M. Rossiter, M.D., *Face Culture.* Pageant Press, Inc., New York, 1956. (Out of print.)

There are various substances you can apply to your face to help wrinkles recede. Sanford Bennett recommended the age-old egg-white mask, which he used regularly. He suggested beating up the white of an egg until frothy, and applying it to the wrinkled areas with a shaving brush. (It is considered safe for under-eye areas if followed with a moisturizer.) Bennett allowed the egg white to remain on his face for five minutes and then rinsed it off with warm water. He used the egg-white treatment daily. Some creams and oils also help. (See chapter ten for these and for helpful exercises for under-eye wrinkles.)

If you wish your face to be your fortune, give it proper care. An example of a woman who believes in face as well as body care for best appearance is Betsy Theodoracopulous. She is thirty-six, has been twice married and has two children. She has been a model for eighteen years. She admits that her good looks and youthful appearance are the result of lots of care. She says, "I get between eight and nine hours of sleep at night. Otherwise, I notice an immediate change in my face.

"I have never had a facial. My skin doctor has told me that in my case it could break down the facial muscles.

"I don't exactly diet, but I eat healthful foods and take vitamins. And so much of the way you look reflects your mental attitude. Even at trying times in my life, I try to keep busy and active and happy, with no chip on my shoulder. That is really the secret."*

**Women's Wear Daily*, March 1972, and *San Francisco Chronicle*, March 13, 1972.

Now for those helpful face exercises. Sanford Bennett wrote, "Exercises . . . if persistently and methodically practiced, will surely restore to an aged body much of the lost strength and elasticity. . . . It is possible in this way to restore to the muscles of age the rounded contour they may have once possessed. But if muscles, especially of the face and neck are neglected, they will present the flabby condition characteristic of old age, even though the rest of the body has been developed through exercise to the strength of an athlete.

"It is therefore necessary to exercise those face muscles just as you have exercised the muscles of the body, and they will surely grow in size, strength and elasticity if so trained. The hollow places in the neck and cheeks can be so filled out, the muscles that surround the eyes can be increased in plumpness . . . and the characteristics of youth, to a very considerable extent, be regained."

In the remaining chapters you will find the all-purpose smile-up exercise, followed by other face exercises, arranged according to each section of the face.

7

THE SMILE-UP EXERCISE

Chapter Seven

The Smile-Up Exercise

The smile-up exercise should be the first and the last exercise in your face-conditioning program every single day. The reason, according to Doctor Rossiter, is that it is a face-lifting exercise.

There are approximately fifty muscles that control your face movements as you express various emotions. On top of these muscles are nerves, tissues and a cushioning layer of fat, which provide facial smoothness and firmness. The entire structure is covered with skin. The muscles usually occur in pairs. Dr. Rossiter said that if you draw an imaginary line, beginning a half-inch away from each corner of your mouth and going upward to a short distance outside the corner of each eye, you have located the laughing muscles. Because these muscles are attached to other muscles, they control most of the muscles of your face.

If you use the smile-up exercise persistently, Dr. Rossiter promised that you will bring about "a permanent, natural lifting of your facial tissues," resulting in a younger-looking and a more pleasant-appearing facial expression. You will look happier and more attractive too, because pleasant emotions and expressions lift the face, whereas depression and anger pull it downward.

Here is the smile-up exercise: Put oil or a heavy night-cream around your eyes to avoid making creases. Press the heels of your hands on the areas on the outside of your eyes to prevent crow's-feet from forming. (Fig. 1) Elevate your chin slightly. Open your mouth about an inch. Lift your upper lip and your check muscles, simultaneously, as in a smile, following the imaginary line you have made of your laughing muscles. Smile upward and squeeze hard. (Fig. 2) Contract your neck muscles, too. Hold to a slow count of six. Relax. Do this exercise ten times.

If you do not believe that this puts your face to work, put your hand on your face, then on the area below your jaw and chin, even on your upper chest near your shoulders while clenching your smile-up. In all, about 100 muscles have been brought into play.

As you relax, increased circulation follows. Your face will feel warm. Dr. Rossiter said, "Remember, it is alternate contraction and relaxation, not stretching, that develops a muscle. This helps to enlarge the muscles more rapidly and permanently lifts the tissues." The muscles also shorten (rather than lengthen and loosen) and become firm. How many times have you been asked to feel the biceps of a man or boy who is proud of his muscles strengthened by body-building exercises or prolonged heavy work? Dr. Rossiter pointed out that, even in repose, these strengthened biceps keep the forearm slightly drawn up. Not only will the smile-up exercise develop, in a similar manner, the uplifting musculature of your face, but your facial muscle tone will improve. Dr. Rossiter stated, "The exercise of the facial muscles definitely improves

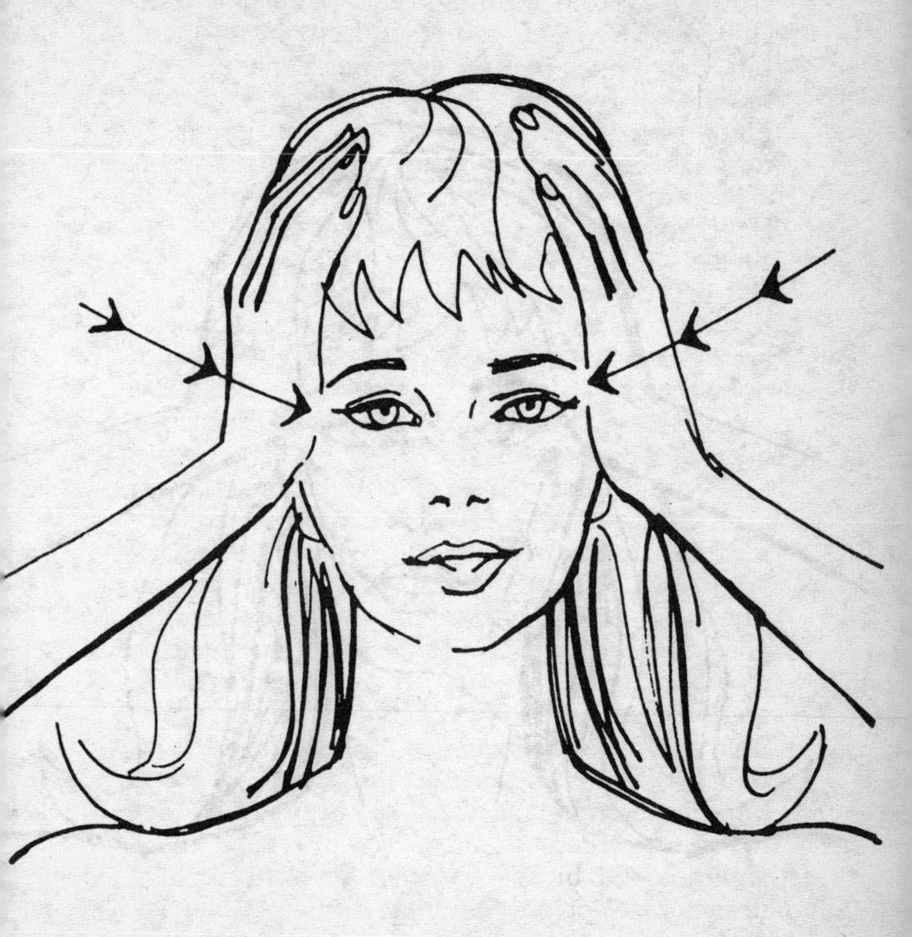

FIG. 1

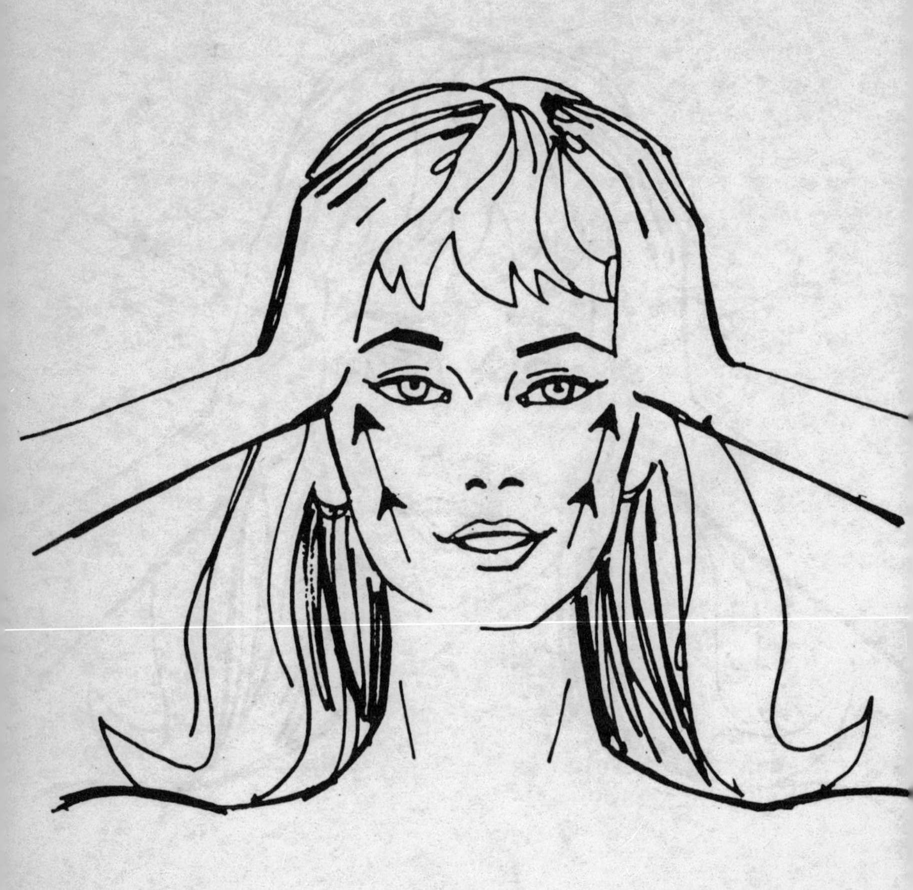

FIG. 2

the tone and appearance of the skin over those muscles. This is a physiological rule."

What did Dr. Rossiter mean by "persistent use" of this exercise? He suggested doing ten smile-up exercises before breakfast, and repeating at intervals throughout the day. He considered twenty to thirty times a day enough at first, but urged working up to at least 100 times a day if possible. If impossible, a few are better than none at all. At first, if your face muscles have become lazy, they may feel sore. But Dr. Rossiter said that this is a good sign that the muscle cells are becoming active and stronger.

How long will it take for results? Dr. Rossiter admitted that the older you are, the slower the results. But, he added, in one week's time you should notice improvement. "Four to six weeks," he said, "will produce permanent changes in your facial expression, changes that will remain even if you stop the exercises for a while. The strengthened muscles will continue to hold your face up." He believed that you would become more enthusiastic about the exercise day after day.

The smile-up is almost a complete all-in-one exercise. However, there are special areas of the face that benefit from special attention to bring even faster results. These exercises appear in the following chapters.

8

YOUR FOREHEAD

Chapter Eight

Your Forehead

Your forehead is controlled by a broad muscle that contains vertical fibers running up and down your forehead from eyebrows to hairline. However, most lines that form on the forehead are horizontal, running from temple to temple. They are not necessarily a sign of aging; they can appear at any age and are caused by nervous lifting, puckering and other unnecessary movements of the forehead while you talk, think or emote. Because there is very little fatty tissue to support the underlying skin on the forehead, smoothing it requires a special method. This method of smoothing your forehead is threefold: re-educating your forehead so that it will remain immobile and serene, even during consternation, surprise or shock; stroking your forehead for relaxation; and exercising the muscles against resistance.

The Exercise

Sit at a table, desk or bathroom countertop, so that you can rest your elbows on a flat surface. Place the palms and heels of both hands, side by side, above your eyebrows. The fingers may touch or overlap slightly as they lie flat on your forehead. For resistance, press your hands

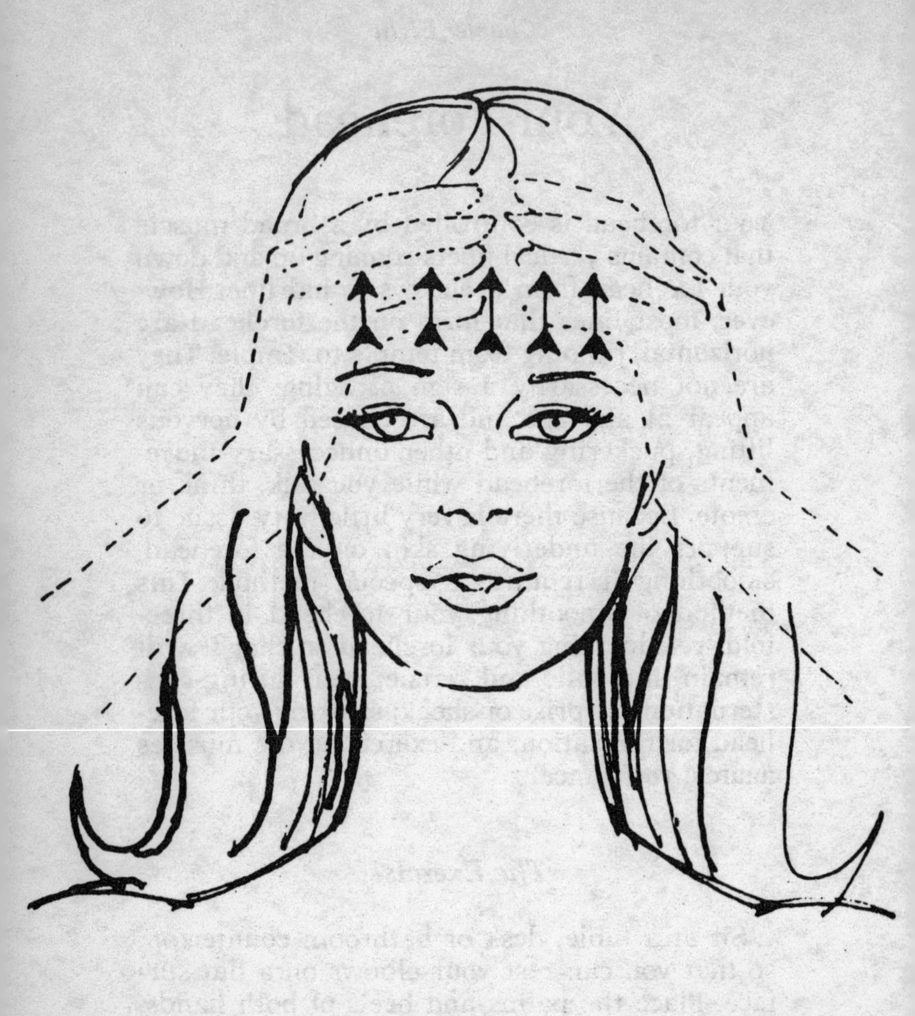

FIG. 3

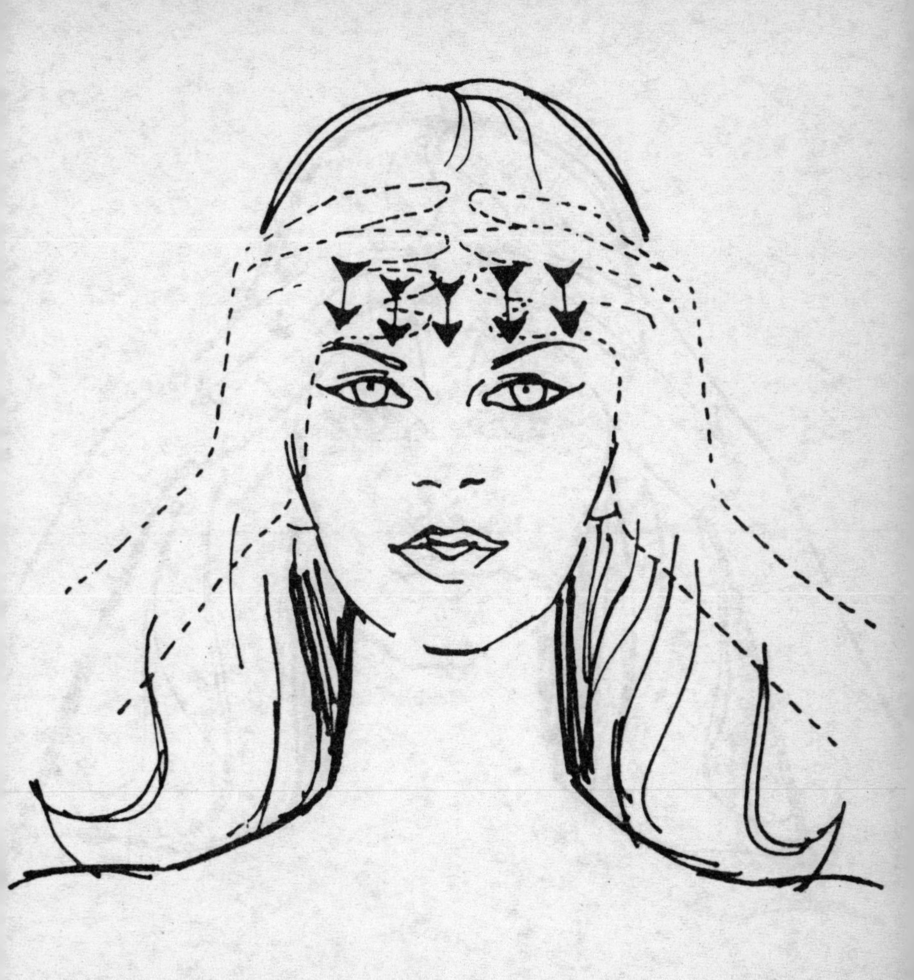

FIG. 4

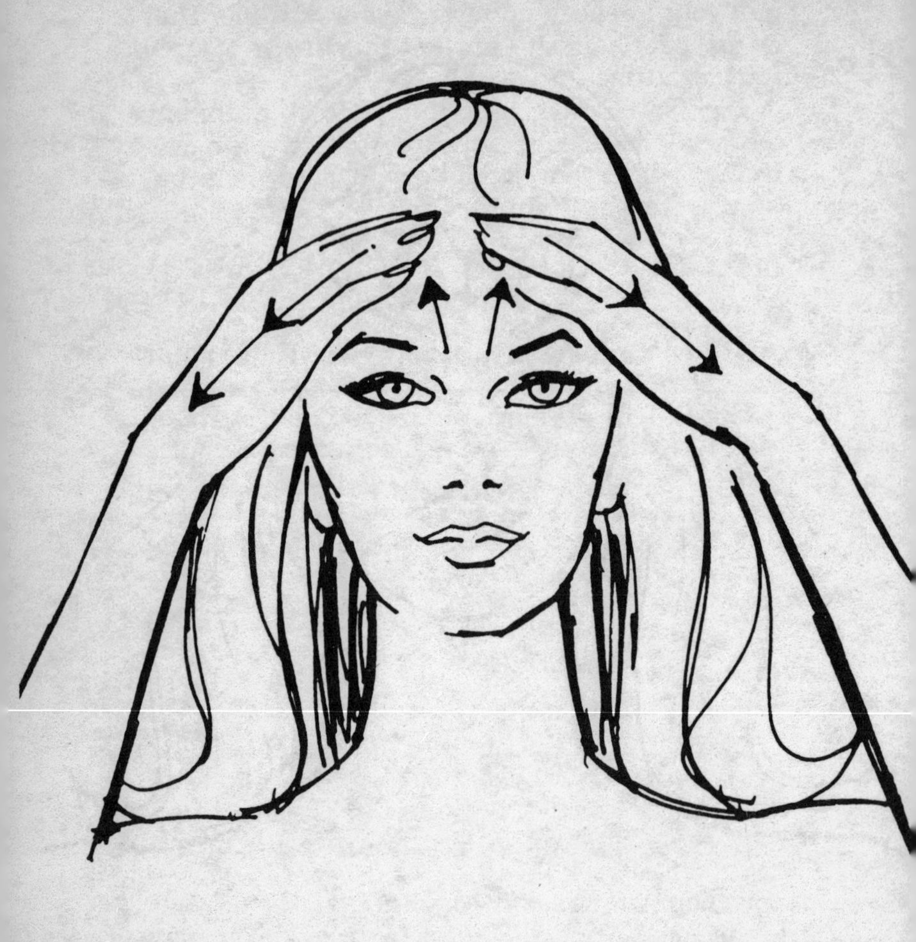

FIG. 5

firmly against your forehead, while you try to pull your forehead up toward your hairline. That is, use your hands to prevent this lifting. (Fig. 3) Repeat 5 times.

Then reverse the procedure. Try to pull your forehead muscles downward toward your eyebrows, while your hands try to hold them up. (Fig. 4) Repeat 5 times.

Stroking

A few people have vertical forehead lines, but stroking helps both types of lines, vertical and horizontal, by encouraging relaxation. Cream or oil your forehead slightly. Resting your elbows on a tabletop, stroke your forehead *gently* with your fingertips, starting from between your brows, in upward and outward, wing-like motions. (Fig. 5) Repeat until you feel a delicious sense of relaxation.

Serenity

A beautiful face is serene, not a series of facial gymnastics. Try always to keep your forehead immobile, so that it will remain placid and serene at all times. Aim first for an hour, then a day, then a week.

To help you break the habit of puckering your forehead as you talk, think and feel, you may apply strips of opaque Scotch tape to the deepest horizontal furrows. The tape will help somewhat to reduce the lines. But, more important, it will remind you to break your habit of unnecessary forehead activity.

9

SCOWL LINES

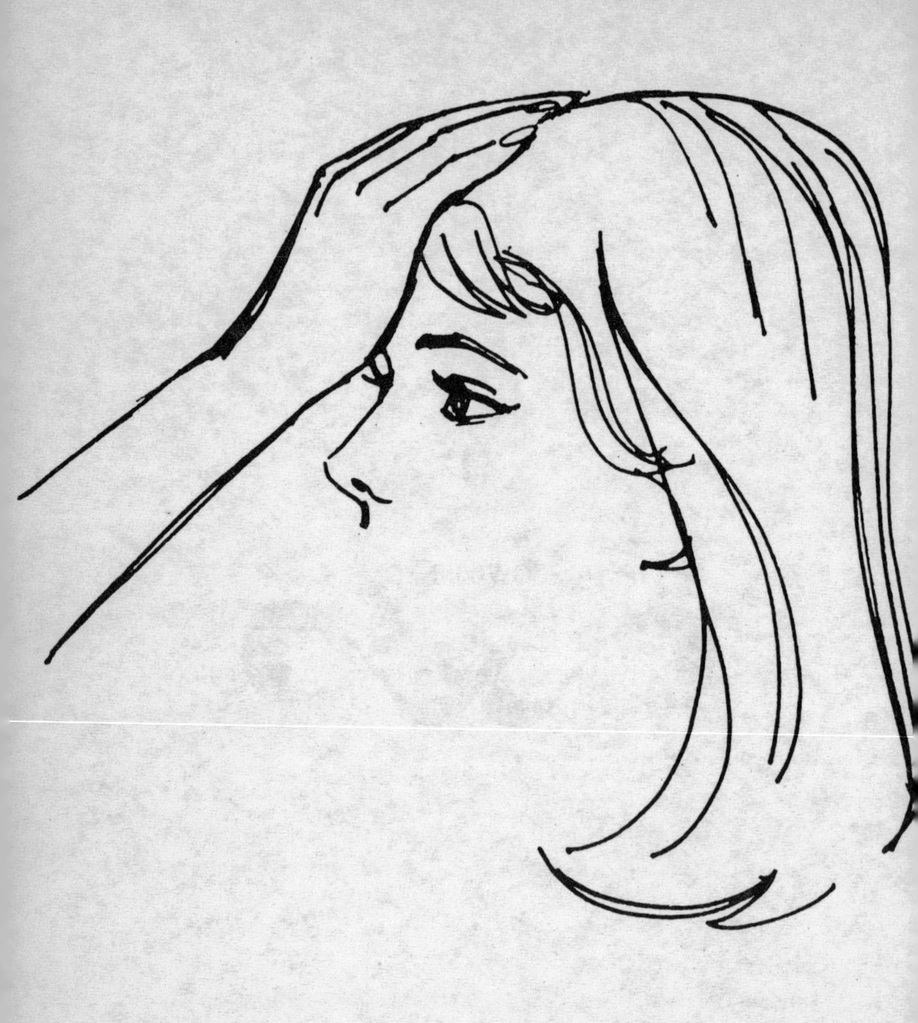

FIG. 6

Chapter Nine

Scowl Lines

There is a little muscle between the eyebrows that extends downward to the top of the nose bone. When this muscle contracts during pain, worry, grief or mental concentration, it creates scowl or frown lines between the eyebrows, and sometimes on the upper bridge of the nose. If the contractions are repeated often enough, the lines may become permanent. The methods of erasing or smoothing these lines are as follows:

Sit in front of a table or another firm surface. Rest your right elbow on the surface if you are right-handed; the left, if you are left-handed. Place the heel of your hand between your eyebrows and press on the scowl lines with the heel of that hand. (Fig. 6) *Make your muscles work against the resistance of your hand pressure* in five separate steps:

1. Pull your frown muscles inward, *toward* the center of your eyebrows, as in frowning, against the firm pressure of your hand. Keep the frowning muscles concentrated tightly for a few seconds. (Fig. 7) Repeat three times, increasing the number daily.

2. Now pull or stretch the frown muscles in the opposite direction, *away* from your eyebrow center, outward toward your ears. As your hand pressure tries to hold back this muscle move-

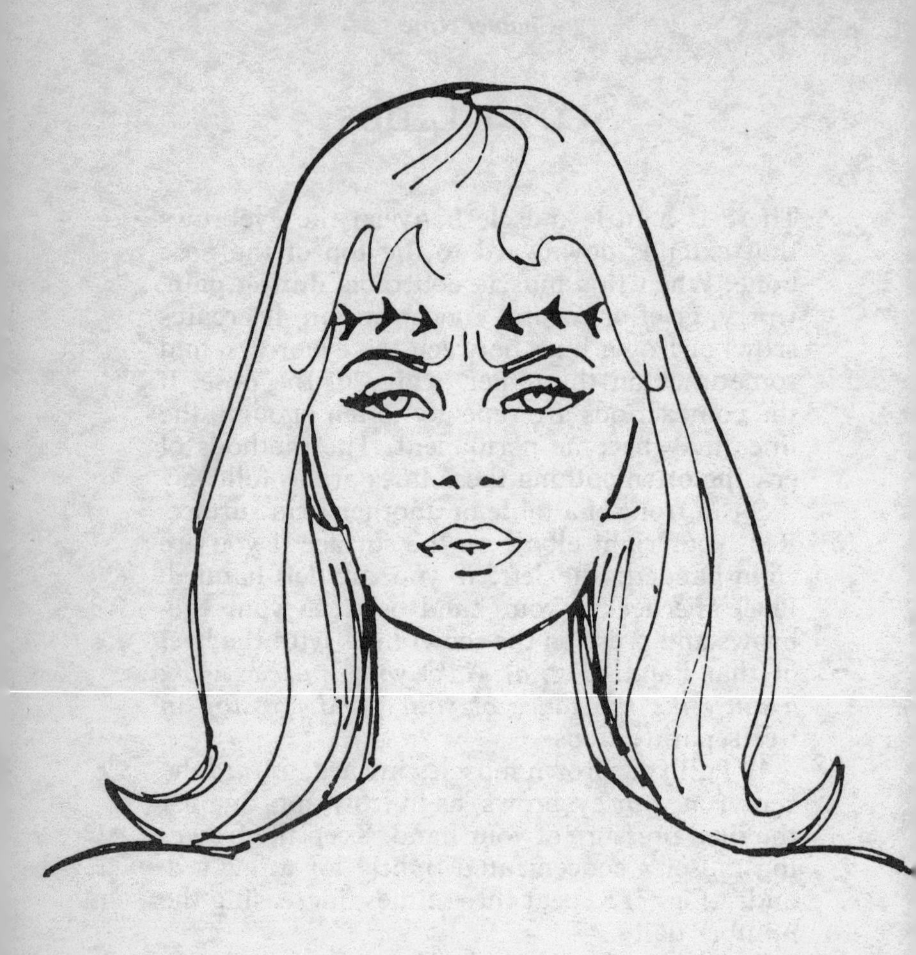

FIG. 7

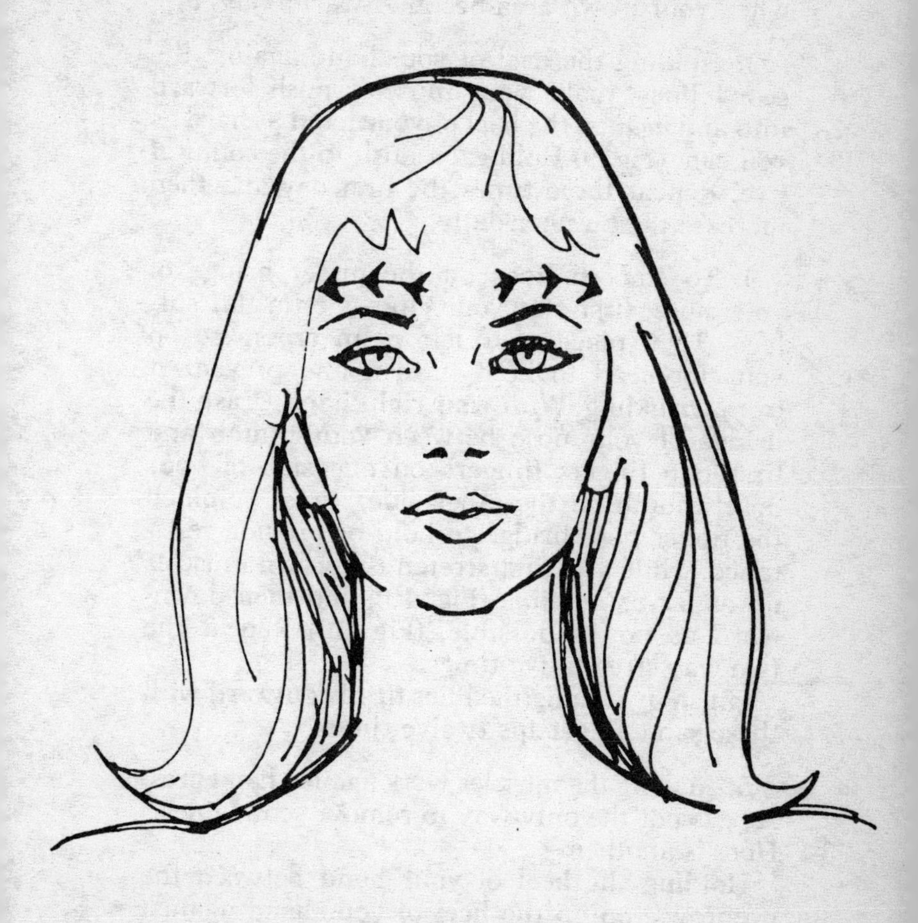

FIG. 8

ment, *make those frown muscles work!* In the beginning, do this exercise three times a day, and increase daily to the point of fatigue, or when your frown area becomes warm. (Fig. 8)

3. Holding the heel of your hand against the scowl lines, make your muscles push forward into and *against* the heel of your hand as hard as you can. (Fig. 9) Hold each push to the count of five. Repeat three times the first day and then increase the number daily.

4. To smooth lines on the upper bridge of your nose, first rest your elbows on a flat surface. Then place your left palm crosswise on your forehead to hold it firm and prevent it from wrinkling. With your right hand, grasp the bridge of your nose between your thumb and first two fingers (fingers on one side of your nose, thumb on the other side). Press or pinch the upper nose bridge to hold or provide resistance, while you first stretch the frown muscles up as far as possible (Fig. 10), and then downward as far as possible. (Fig. 10) Repeat the two-way stretch five times.

Finish by ironing the lines firmly outward with these same fingertips twelve times.

5. Making the muscles work against hand pressure is not the only way to remove scowl lines. Here is another:

Holding the heel of your hand between the eyebrows, pump the heel of your hand against your scowl lines, in and out, in and out, to create suction and plump out the tissues lying beneath your hand. This is an extremely benefi-

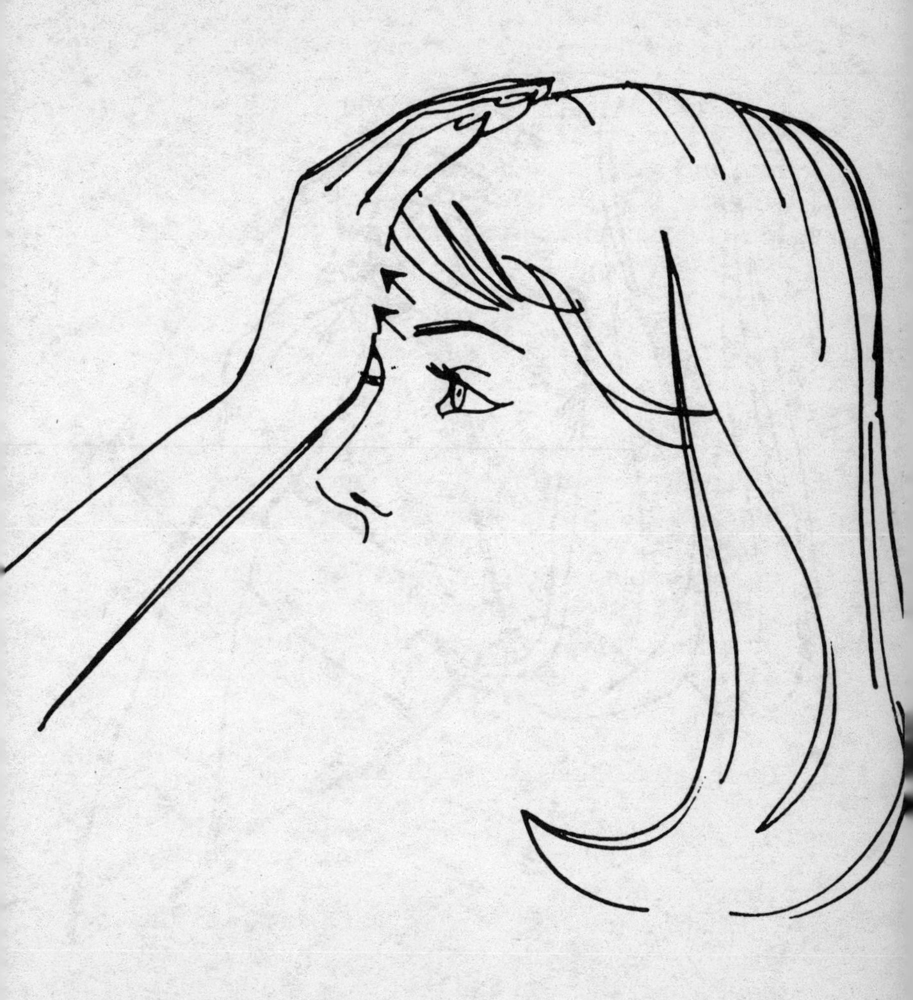

FIG. 9

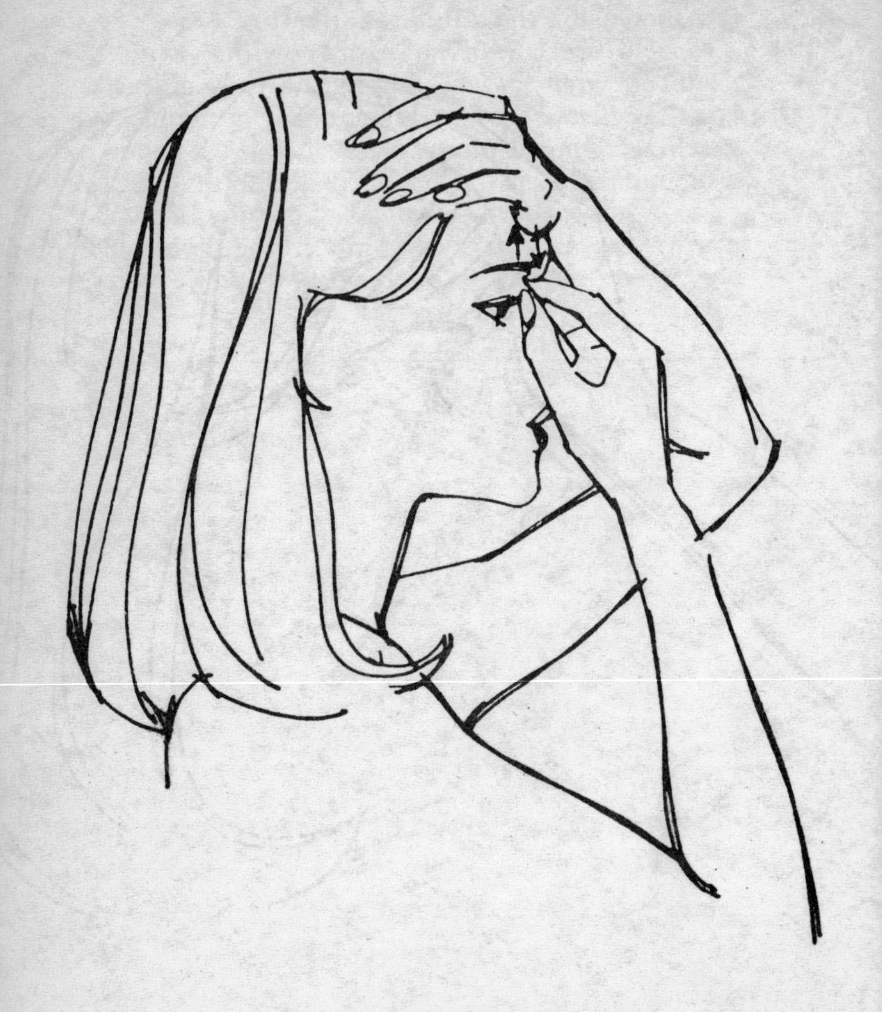

FIG. 10

cial exercise to improve circulation, plump tissues and smooth lines. Start with ten times a day, increasing the number daily. (Fig. 11)

To help break your habit of scowling (which produced your frown lines in the first place), wear the little devices known as "Frownies," which are shaped pieces of flesh-colored paper with mucilage on the back (available at drugstores). Or apply crossed strips of opaque Scotch tape to keep new furrows from forming. You can wear these devices as you work or while you sleep.

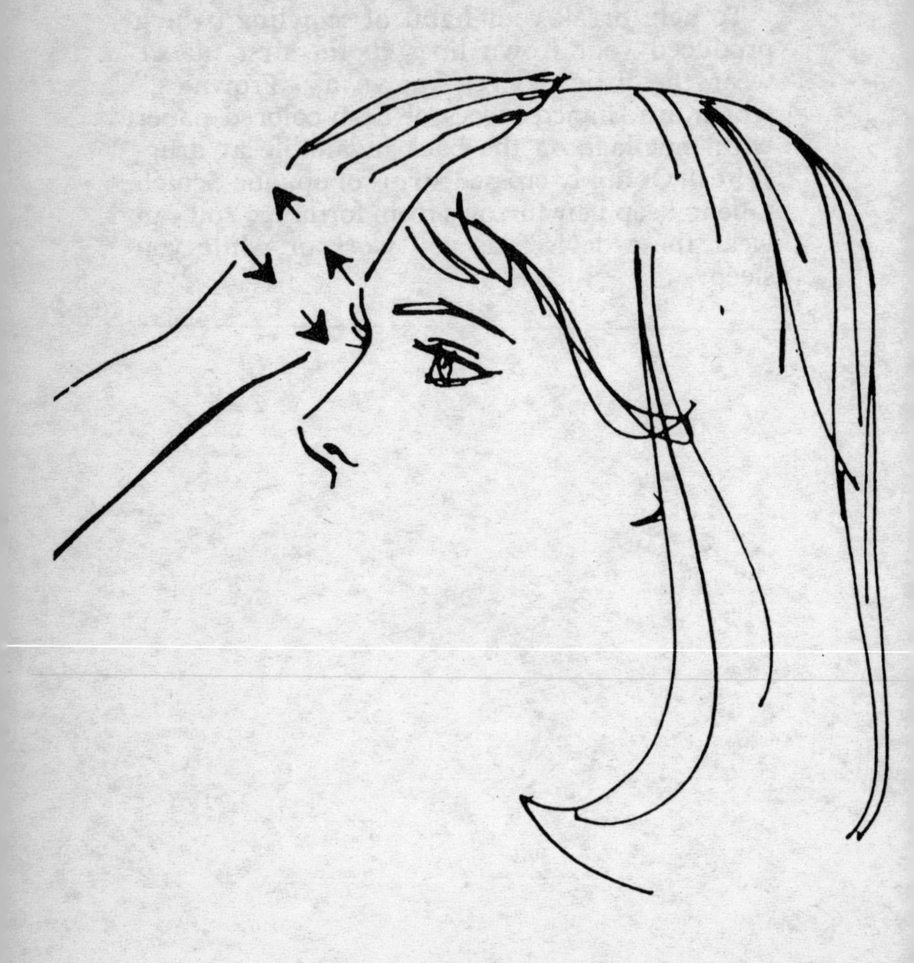

FIG. 11

10

YOUR EYES

Chapter Ten

Your Eyes

Here are some exciting and helpful methods of dealing with eye area beauty problems.

Do as many of your eye exercises as possible on the slant board. Jheri Redding, beauty expert, says, "Often the simple procedure of lying for fifteen minutes on a slant board will greatly reduce droopy under-eye tissue and aid in diminishing those fine lines that accompany the baggy droop. Whatever cream or oil you put on your face is absorbed more readily in a slant position. Masques are also more beneficial à la slant board."

Jheri Redding suggests this exercise to improve crinkly lines under the eyes as well as any puffiness that may be present:

"Lying on the slant board, place two fingertips of the left hand on the top of the left cheekbone, and pull down, toward your body. Try to close your left eye, but exert enough resistance with your fingertips to prevent the eye from actually closing. (Fig. 12) Count to six slowly while still attempting to close your eye against the resisting pull of your fingertips. Repeat with your right eye. A count of six is enough."

Mr. Redding also recommends the use of a home-made cream to apply under and around your eyes as follows: Combine one ounce of col-

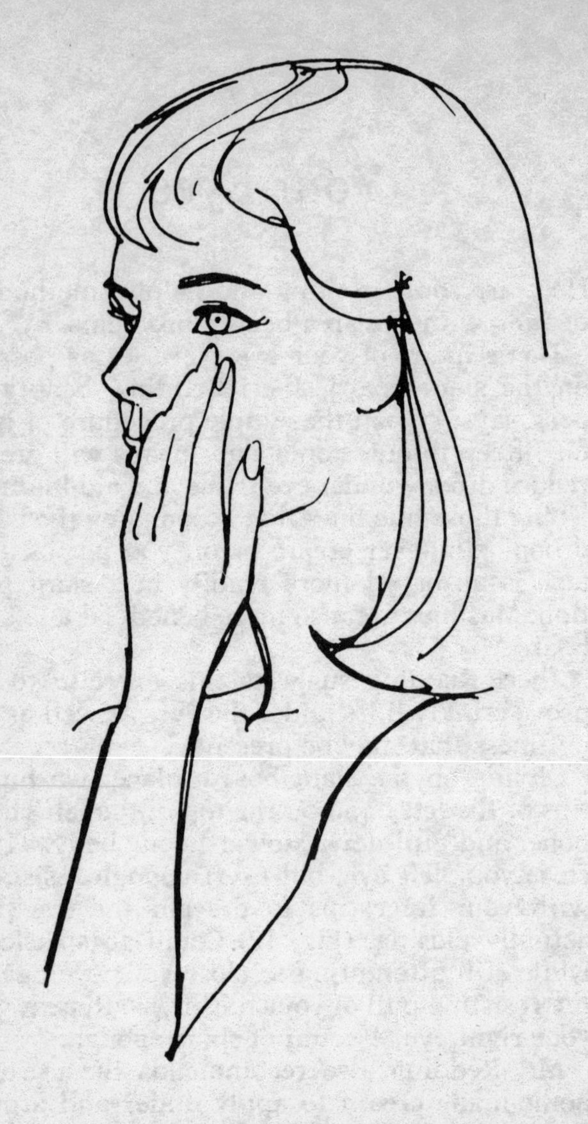

FIG. 12

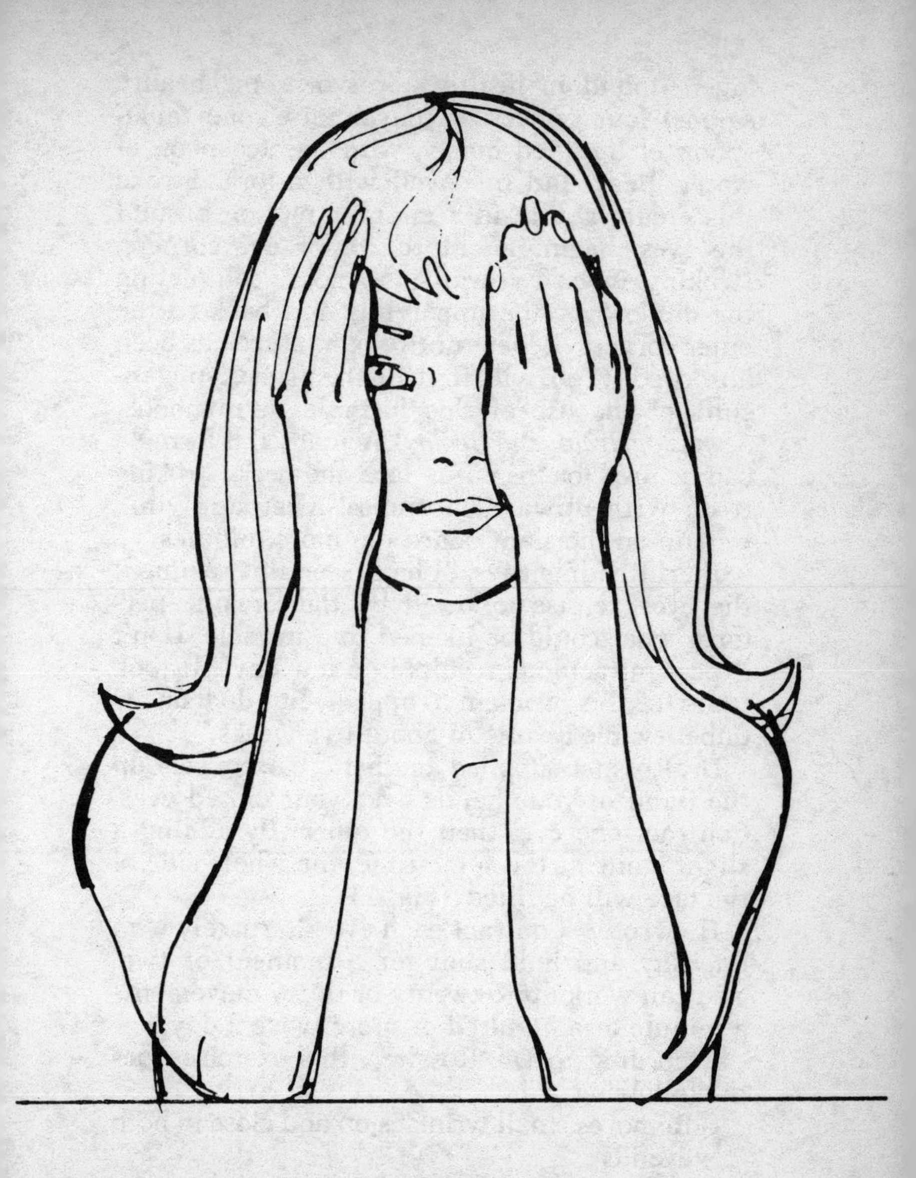

FIG. 13

lagen (found in health stores or some beauty salons) four ounces of mayonnaise, one tablespoon of liquified honey, with one teaspoon of water. Beat, and mix well with a fork. Stroke this cream gently in a circular motion around the eyes, beginning at the outer eye corners, stroking inward toward the nose, completing the circle over the upper lids and back to the outer corners. Repeat until the mixture has been absorbed. (You will find further surprising results of the use of this formula in my book, *Secrets of Health and Beauty*). Actually this formula can be used for the entire face and neck (stroking it on with upward motions). After applying, remain on the slant board ten more minutes.

Jheri Redding says, "I have seen this regimen: the eye exercise followed by the 'cream,' perform what could be likened to a miracle. Don't expect miraculous results in a few days. It took years for this problem to appear. But do look for unbelievable results in about five weeks."

Dr. Rossiter supplied another eye exercise: Cup the palm of your hands over your closed eyes. Contract one eye, then the other. By adding a slight smile at the same time, the whole side of the face will be lifted. (Fig. 13)

He wrote, "Contract each eye alternately *with intensity* and hold shut for a moment or two. You can work up to twenty or thirty movements a minute or a hundred or more twice a day."

According to Dr. Rossiter, this exercise does the following:

—Removes small wrinkles on and close to both eyelids

—Helps prevent bags under the eyelids

—Helps remove dark circles from under the eyes

—Adds tone to the lids and a more vital expression to the eyes

And if you close both eyes tightly at the same time it will also help remove horizontal forehead lines.

Finally, here are strengthening exercises for all muscles involved in and surrounding the eyes, to increase circulation and help tighten flabby tissues and skin lines. These exercises should be repeated just to the point of fatigue, increasing the count daily.

1. Cup your palms over your closed eyes (as in Fig. 13). Tense your eye muscles by contracting or squeezing them tightly.

2. Cupping the bony structure around your eyes firmly with your palms, but without pressing on the eyes themselves, try to move the eye muscles against resistance, first upward, then downward. Repeat this two-way stretch. (Figs. 14 and 15)

3. Now (and this requires concentration), while still cupping your eyes, stretch the eye muscles toward the *outer* eye edges (Fig. 16), then return them to center.

To help correct droopy eyelids—repeat stretching eyelids *upward* and *outward*. Hold to a slow count of six. (Fig. 17)

4. Cupping the eye area firmly with your palms, as before, try to rotate or pull your *under-eye* muscles toward the center, or toward your nose, to strengthen them. (Fig. 18)

5. Holding your palms as a suction cup pressed tightly against the bony ridges around your eyes,

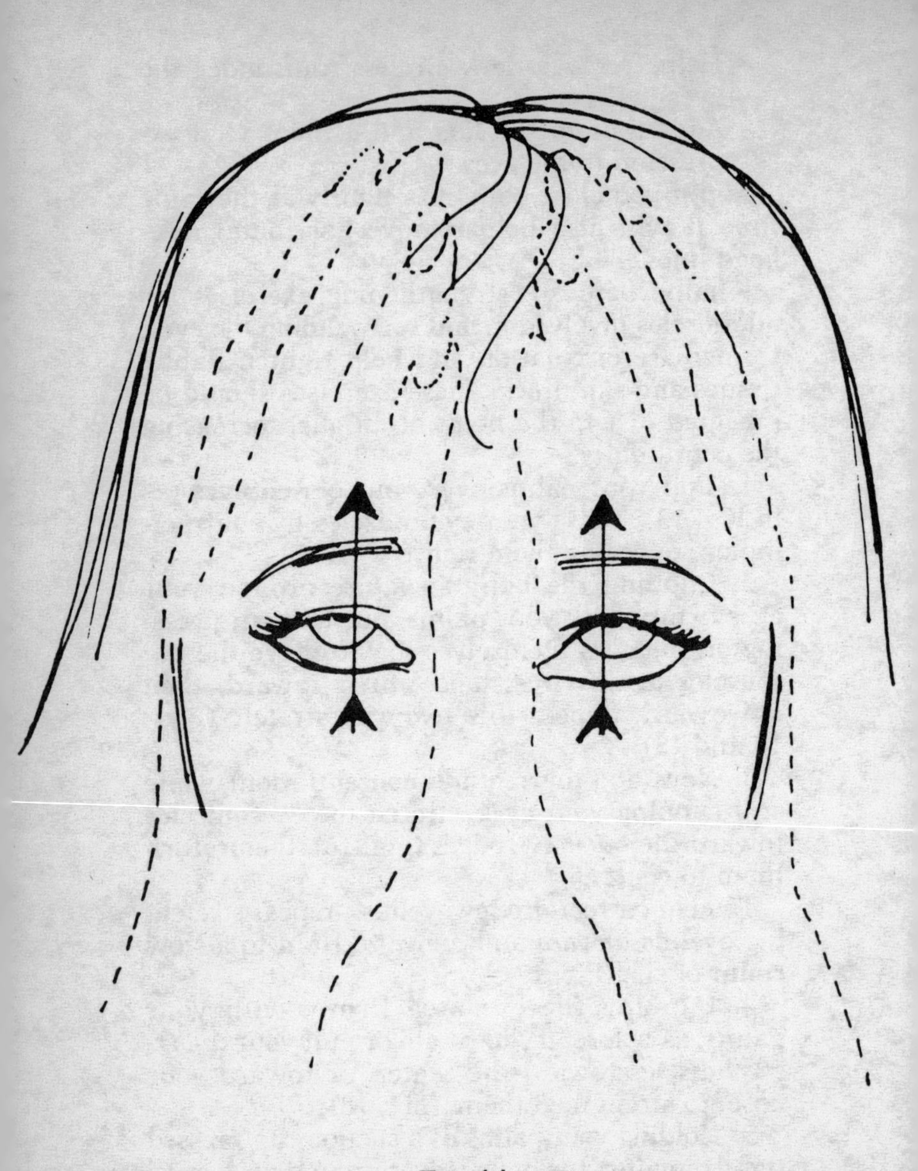

FIG. 14

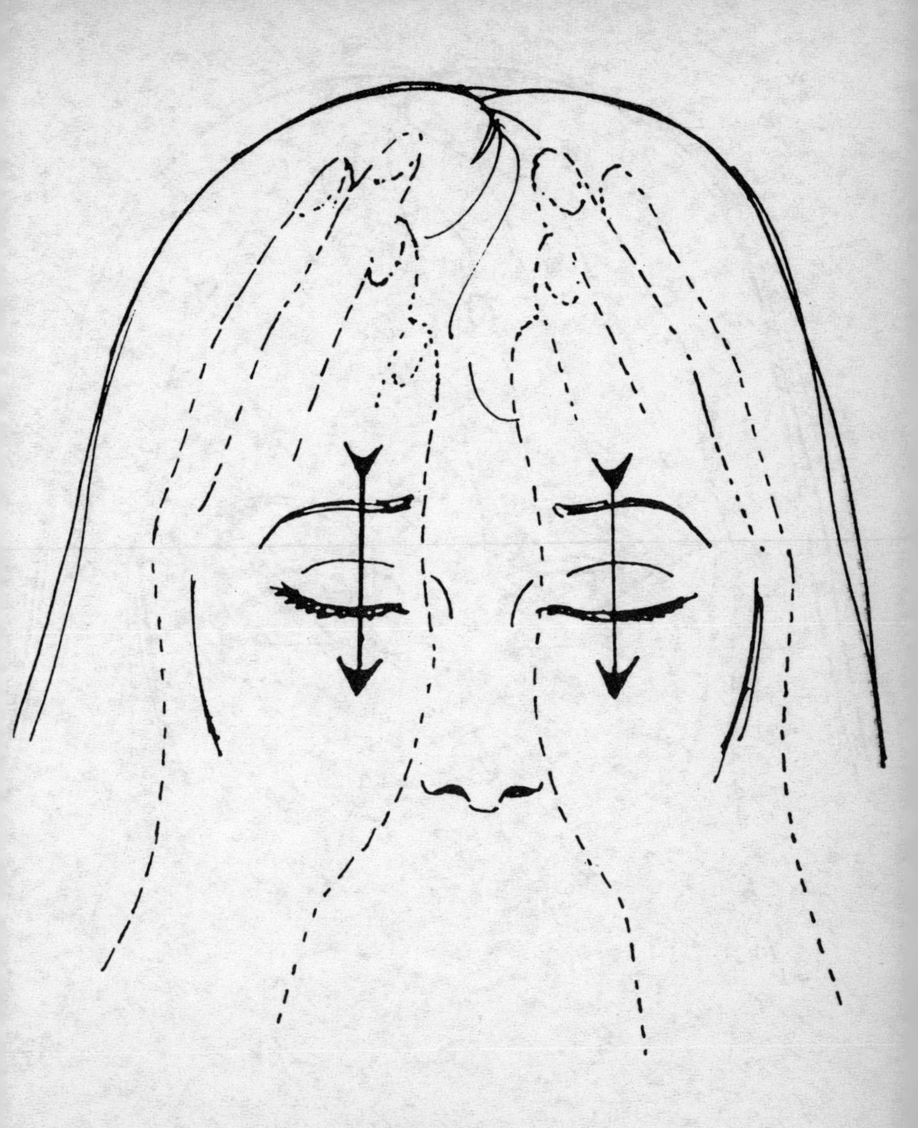

FIG. 15

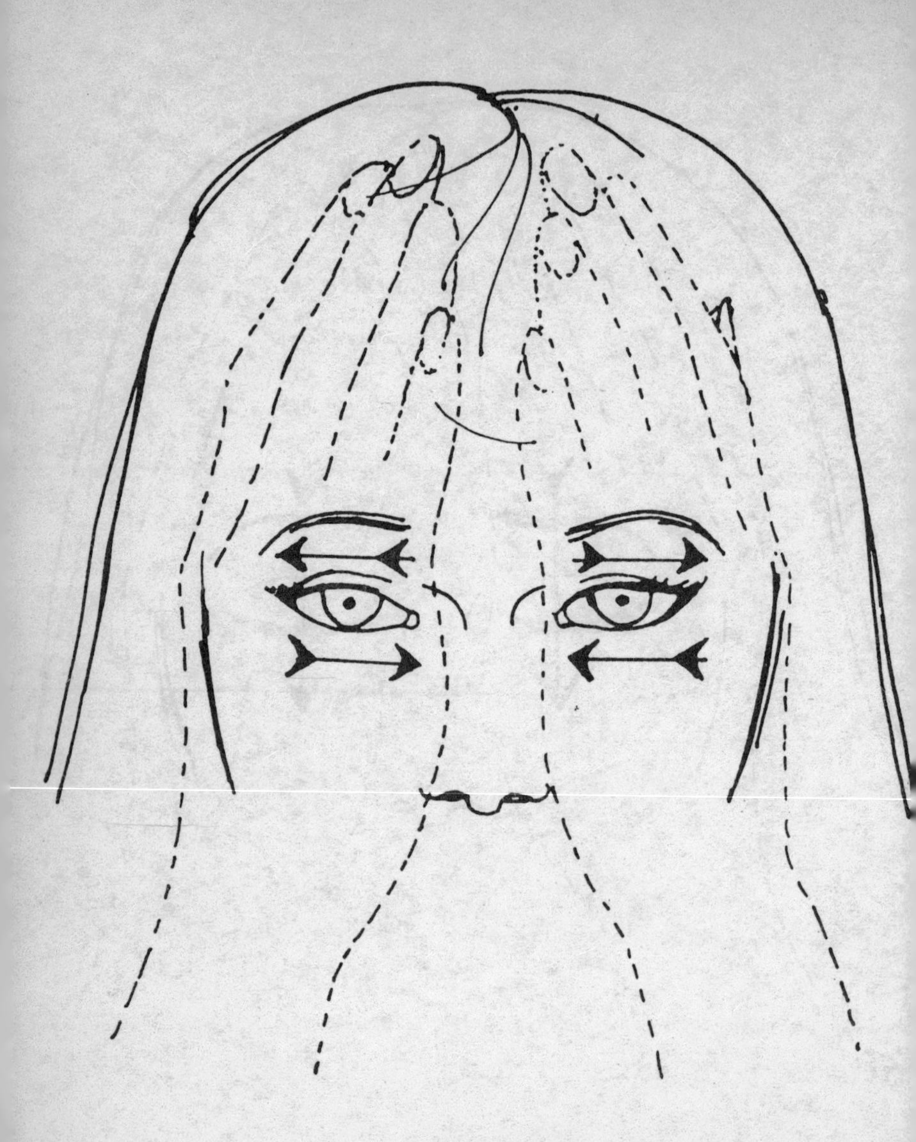

FIG. 16

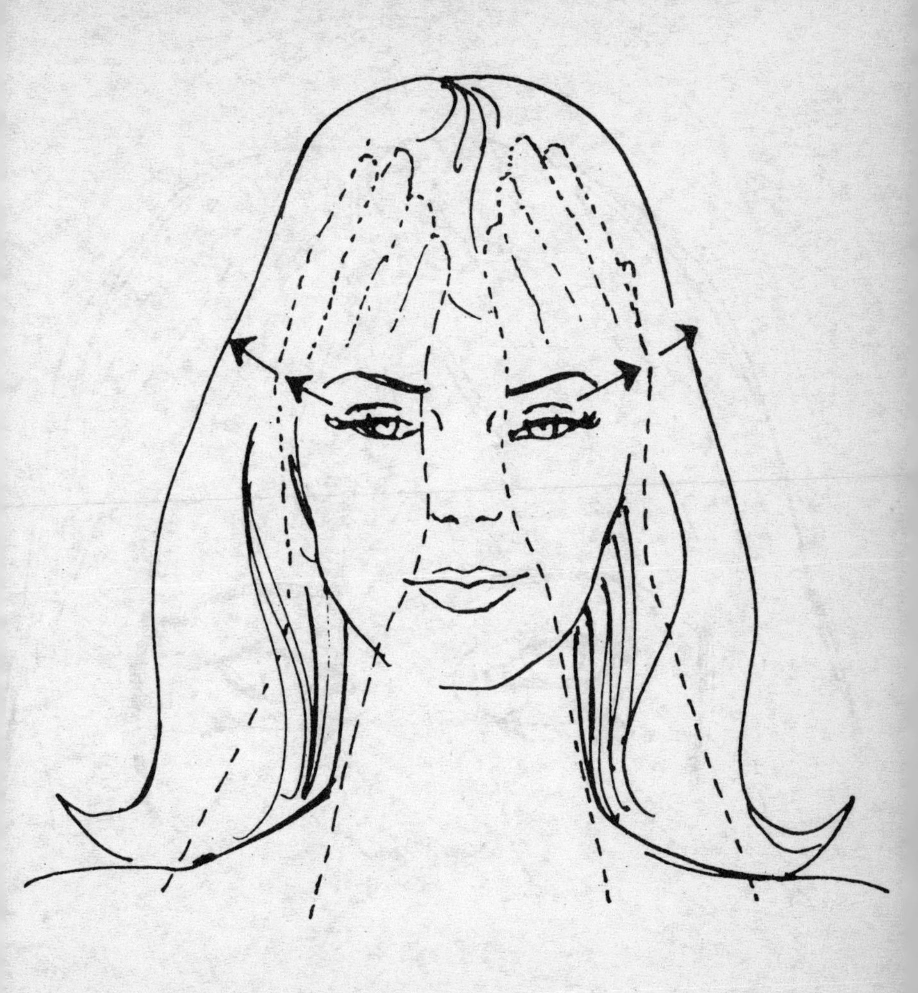

FIG. 17

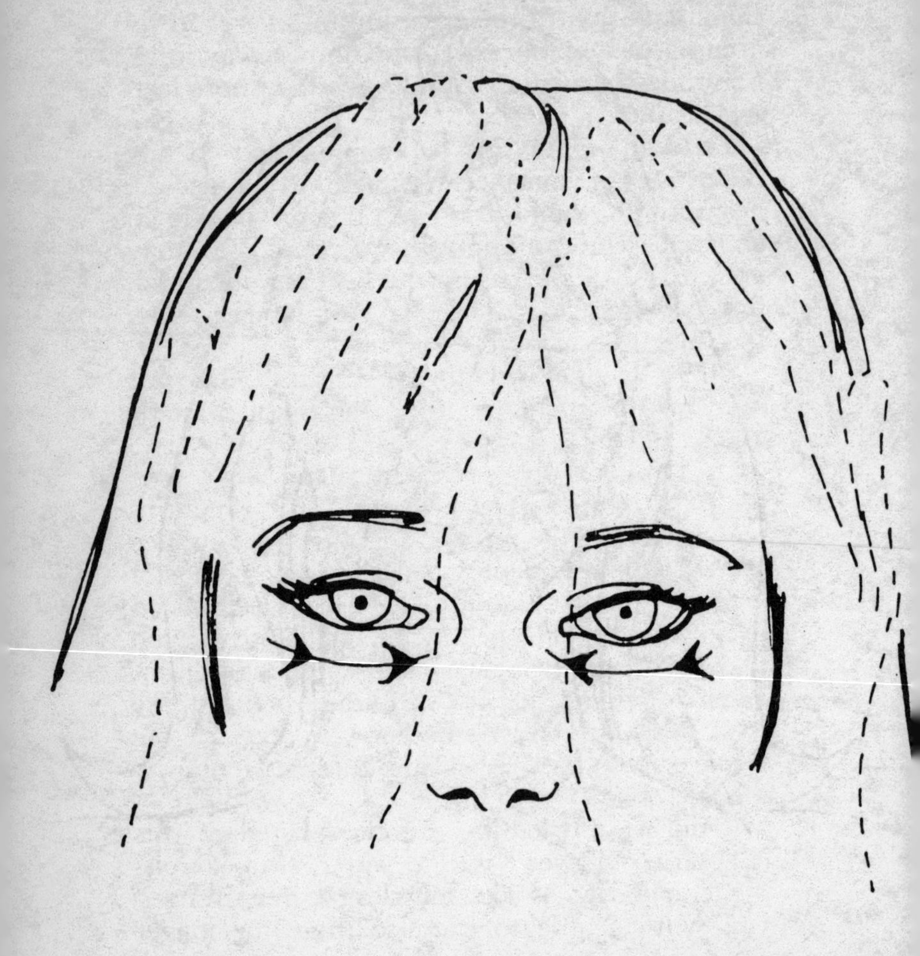

FIG. 18

and without lifting your hands from your skin, create a suction or pumping motion: push and pull, push and pull (Fig. 19) This exercise draws the circulation to the area and inflates the eye-area tissues temporarily, smoothing away lines. Continued use will eventually produce more lasting results.

You can apply this suction method to any other lines in your face. You will have to decide, according to the location of a line or wrinkle on your face, how to apply this method. You may get best results by using the heel of your hand, fingertip, fingertips or even an entire finger across the line, if necessary.

There is one warning to observe. Do not over-do! This suction method undeniably plumps up the tissue beneath the line, but if you overdo it, it may possibly bruise the tissue. Easy does it! At first the effect is temporary. But if continued regularly, the method may help to produce more lasting results provided, as in any method of wrinkle removal, the wrinkles are not reinduced by grimacing or other facial bad habits. Even though at first the results seem to be temporary, wherever circulation is continually induced, the tissues benefit. This is a secret of encouraging tissue repair used by some European physiotherapists.

If during any of the exercises listed in this chapter, your eyes begin to water, stop exercising temporarily. As your muscles become stronger, you will be able to exercise them for longer periods.

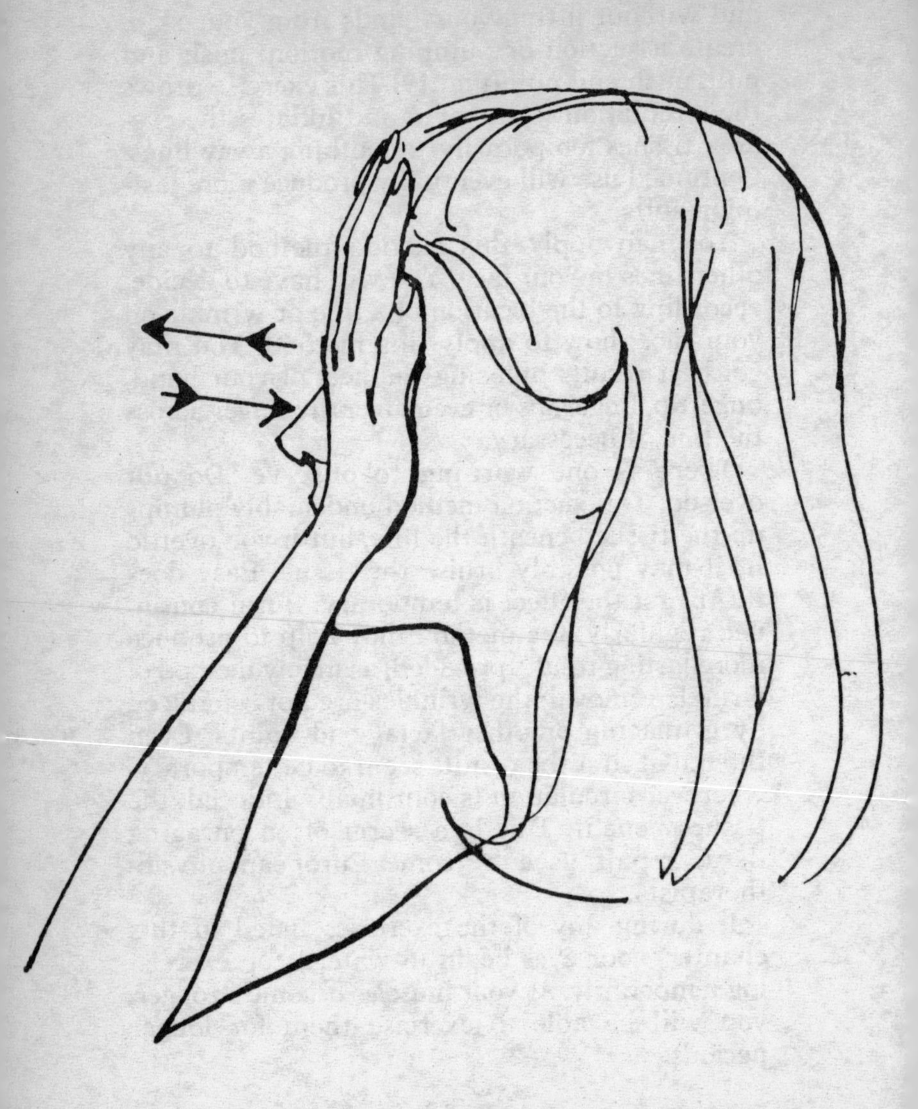

FIG. 19

11

ABOUT LINES

Chapter Eleven

Parenthesis and Sunburst Lines

Most facial conditions respond to the smile-up exercise. However, there are several special problems that may need additional help.

Parenthesis Marks

For parenthesis marks, on either or both sides of your nose, treat one side at a time. Lay your third (your longest) finger against the parenthesis mark for resistance. Smile slightly and tense the muscle underlying the finger and parenthesis. Tense *hard* and relax. Tense and relax until the area becomes warm. Repeat on the other side of your face if necessary. (Fig. 20)

Suck in both cheeks as much as possible. Pull one side of your face toward the opposite side, tense the parenthesis area on the other side, and hold for a count of six seconds, slowly thinking, "one and a two and a three," etc. (Fig. 21)

A tensing, stationary, holding exercise, compared to an active exercise (repeated over and over) is known as an isometric exercise. Both kinds of exercises stir up faster circulation, but

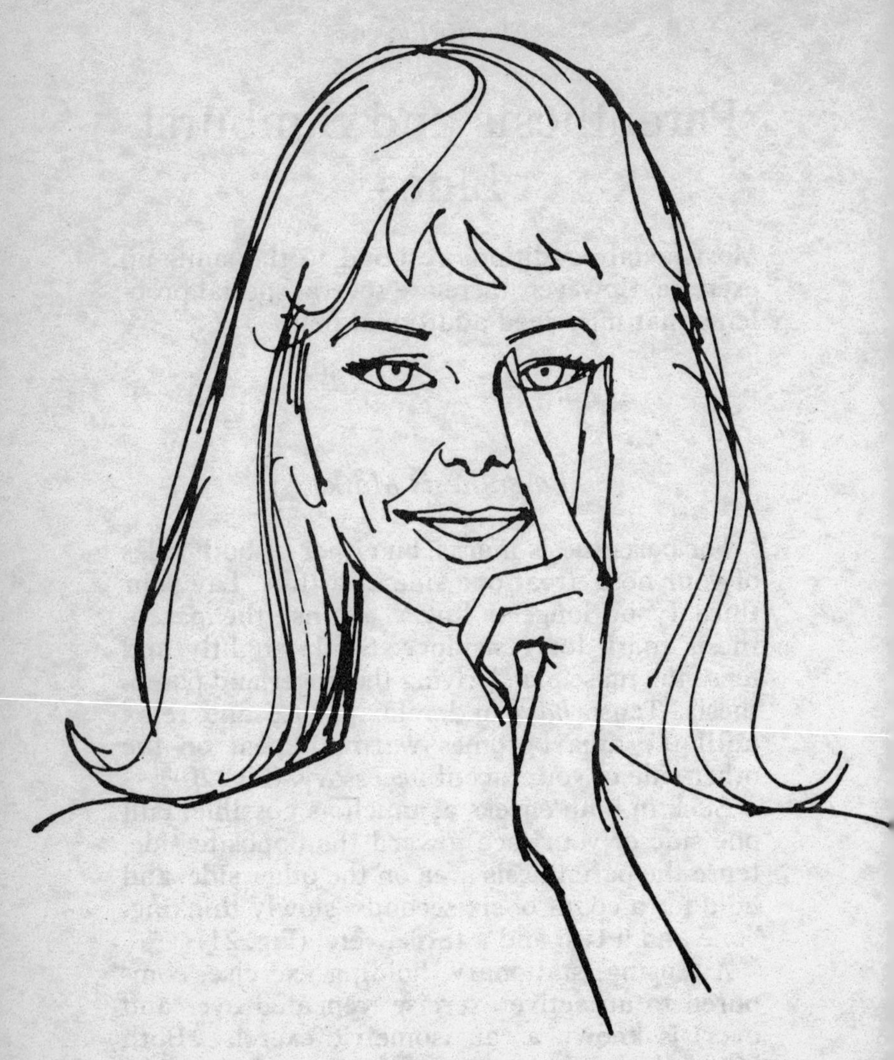

FIG. 20

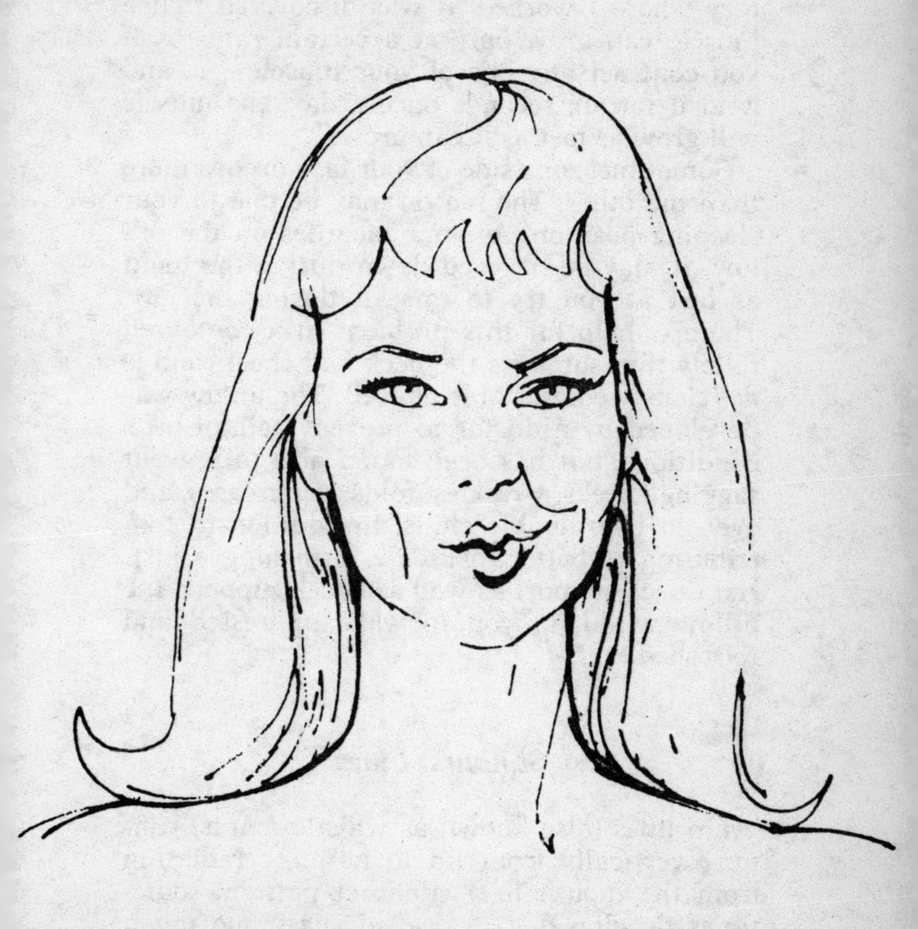

FIG. 21

the isometrics have value for a different reason. A college professor of physiology, Dr. A. H. Steinhaus, explains why: "In a German laboratory where I worked, it was discovered that a muscle can grow only at a certain rate. . . . If you contract any one of your muscles . . . and hold it for six seconds once a day, the muscle will grow as fast as it can grow."

Sometimes, one side of your face droops more than the other. The reason may be due to your sleeping position. As your face lies on the pillow, it may be dragged down during the night as fast as you try to raise it during the day. There is help for this problem in a contoured pillow that supports the neck and cheek, and is deliciously comfortable as well. The pillow was developed by a doctor to prevent painful neck conditions, but has been found also to prevent sagging cheeks, wrinkles, folds and creases, and even to help double chins. In addition to contributing to better looks, by furnishing a just-right neck support as well as cheek support, the pillow will help you to wake up rested and refreshed.*

Sunburst Lines

Lip lines (also known as whistle marks) running vertically from lip to nose, or radiating from the mouth in a sunburst pattern, sometimes develop due to deep dryness, too much

---

*For pillow information, write Patricia Allison Beauty Sorority, Box 1680, La Jolla, Calif. 92037.

sun, chemical depilatories, wearing dentures, or just plain muscle weakness. Dr. Rossiter suggested an exercise for this problem. Insert the first joint of each index finger as a hook inside each corner of the mouth. Smile slightly. Try to stretch your mouth toward your ears with your hooked fingers, as you resist the pull with your mouth itself. (Fig. 22) Exercise to the point of fatigue.

While you are exercising your mouth, you are also exercising twenty other muscles. For example, Dr. Rossiter explained, "No one can smile with separated lips and teeth without contracting the muscles under the chin and jaw." He said that it was his own lip lines that started him on this system of facial rehabilitation. He began the mouth exercise and the smile-up exercise with vigor. He said, "I retired at night with a sore, tired mouth, and aching face, jaw and neck muscles."

At the end of seven days he reported definite improvement which was noticed by others; in a month, the lines and crevices around his mouth had become fuller and firmer.

An excellent alternating isometric exercise to add is as follows:

Make an "O" of your mouth. Holding the mouth tense for resistance, feel the muscles which radiate outward as in a sunburst pattern, pulling *hard*. Hold for a count of six seconds. (Fig. 23) Repeat until the area feels warm. This exercise, too, encourages circulation, strengthens the muscles surrounding your mouth, helps to plump up the tissues, firm the lips and eradicate lip lines. Try it and see!

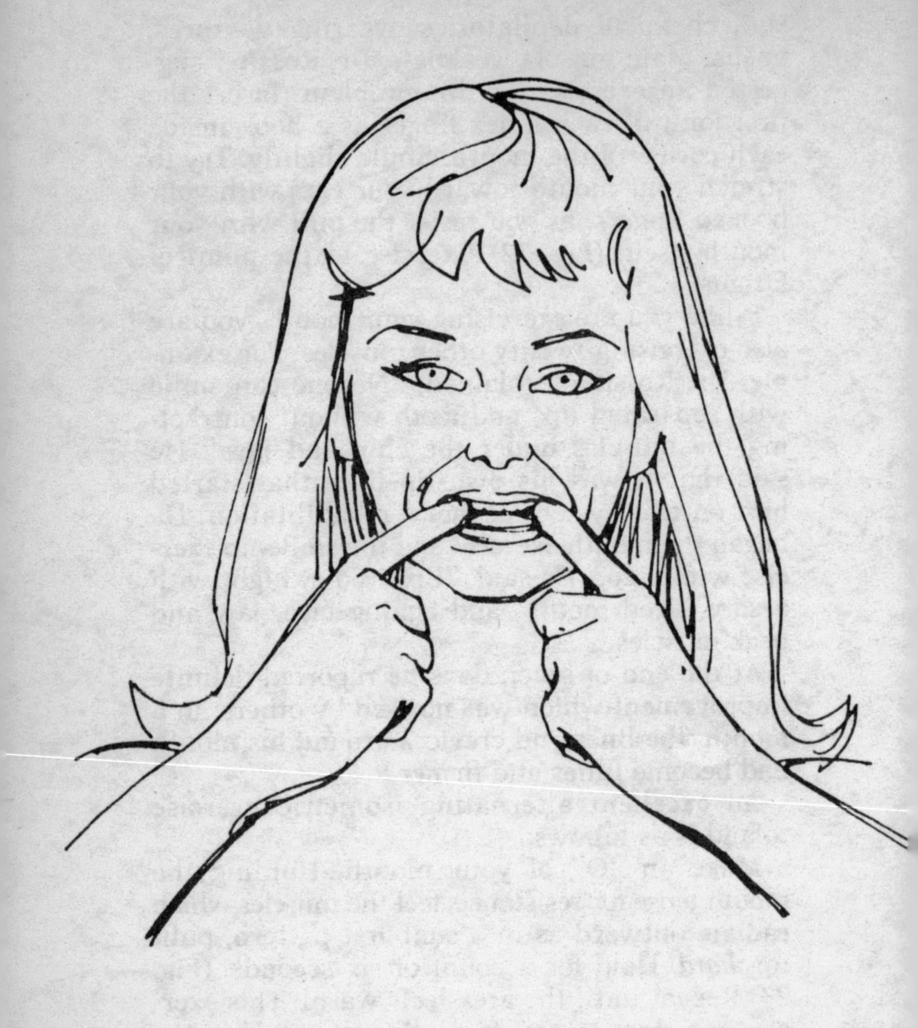

FIG. 22

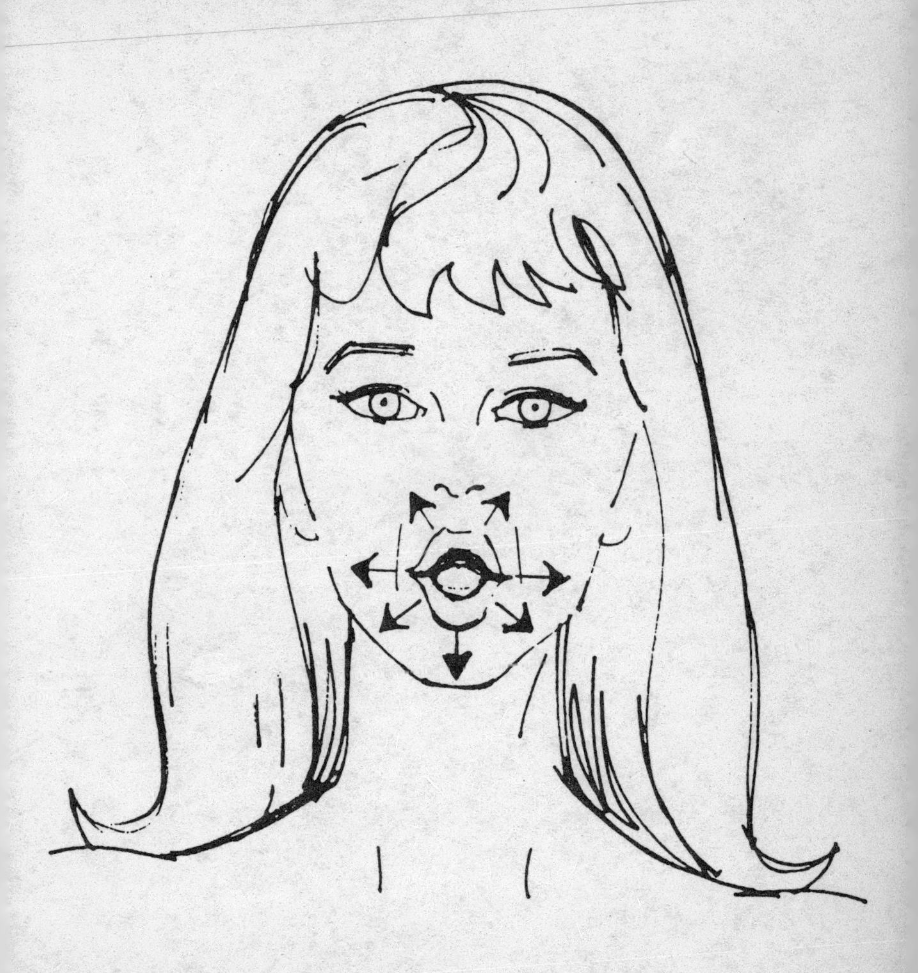

FIG. 23

12

YOUR NECK

Chapter Twelve

Your Neck

The first telltale signs of aging usually appear in the neck. They may be partly due to poor diet, poor circulation, weakened neck muscles, the pull of gravity and poor posture. Ballet dancers who have excellent posture and, directly or indirectly, exercise their neck muscles as they practice and perform their art, often maintain a swan-like neck into a much later age than others. If you stretch the back of your neck upward to lengthen it, you automatically pull your ears back, pull up the muscles of both the back and the front of the neck and encourage stronger muscles and better circulation. Just by feeling that the top of your head is being pulled upward, and by stretching up the back of your neck, you will almost instantaneously improve your frontal neck area. Native girls of various tribes who carry baskets and other weights on their heads, hold their heads high and their necks straight. Members of royalty are trained to do the same thing for appearance's sake. Stand straight and stretch your neck back and upward always. Not only will you look better and more regal, but you will feel better. Try it!

Look at the people you see on the street. Instead of carrying their heads aloft, they allow gravity to produce a shoulder slump; their head vard, far out of line with their . Result: a crumpled front-neck dowager's hump, and always a pearance. Fortunately there are corxercises both to help your neck mus- y gravity and to improve the appearance your neck. Many people have reported transforming a sagging neck into a more youthful-looking one. The sooner the problem is attacked (or prevented), the faster and more successful the results. In any event, you *can* improve your neck through the following exercises.

As a researcher and reporter, I believe I own every book and pamphlet ever published on the subject of face and neck exercises. There are not a great many of them (approximately ten or so), but most of them have given, in one form or another, the following exercise for neck improvement. Patricia Allison, who supplies natural cosmetics that contain no chemicals at all, calls her version "Star's Secret":

"Lie on your back across the bed. Shoulders should be supported by the bed. Neck and head should hang backward limply over the edge of the bed. Completely relax all tensions. (Fig. 24) Inhale and exhale deeply. Now *slowly* raise head, chin first, until your chin touches your chest. (Fig. 25) Then *slowly* (this provides necessary resistance) lower head back to limp, hanging position. Inhale, exhale. Repeat. Two counts are sufficient for a beginner. Work up to six counts every morning."

Dr. Rossiter's version of this same exercise is done in an upright position, tensing the head as

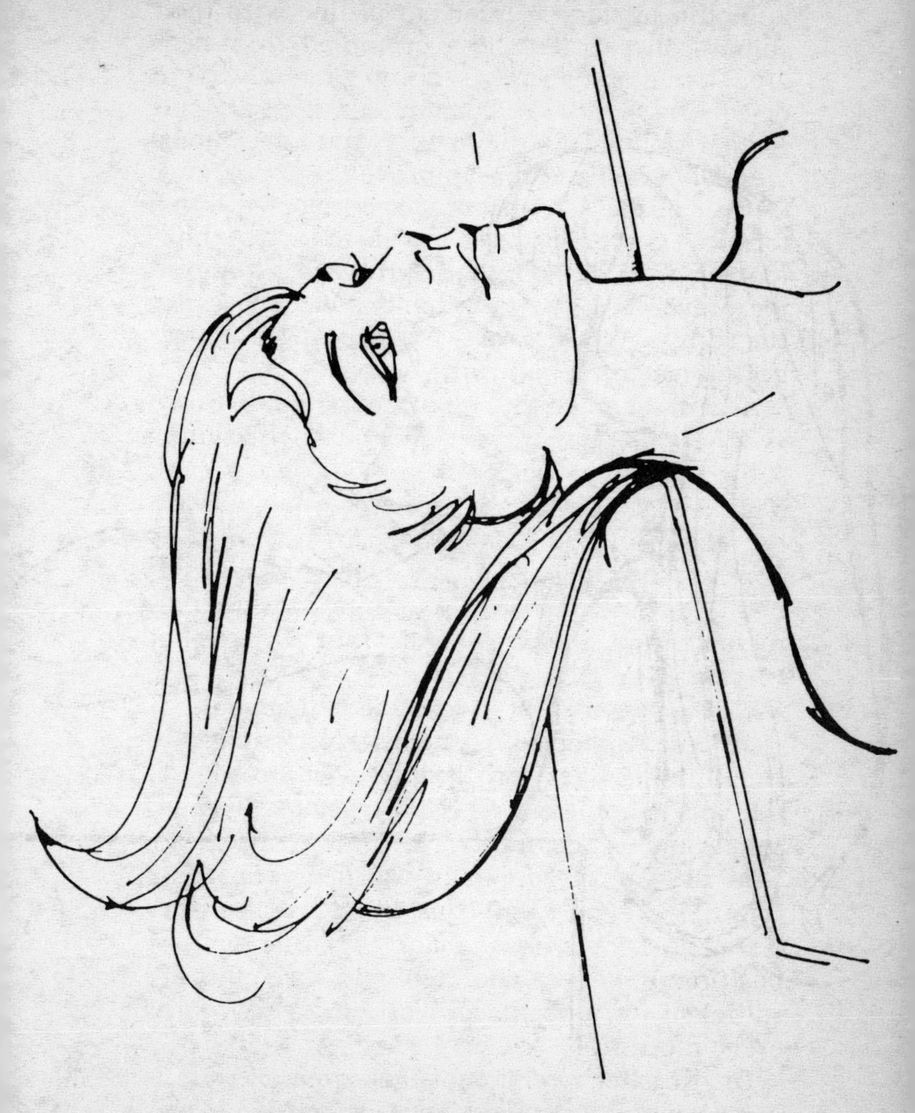

FIG. 24

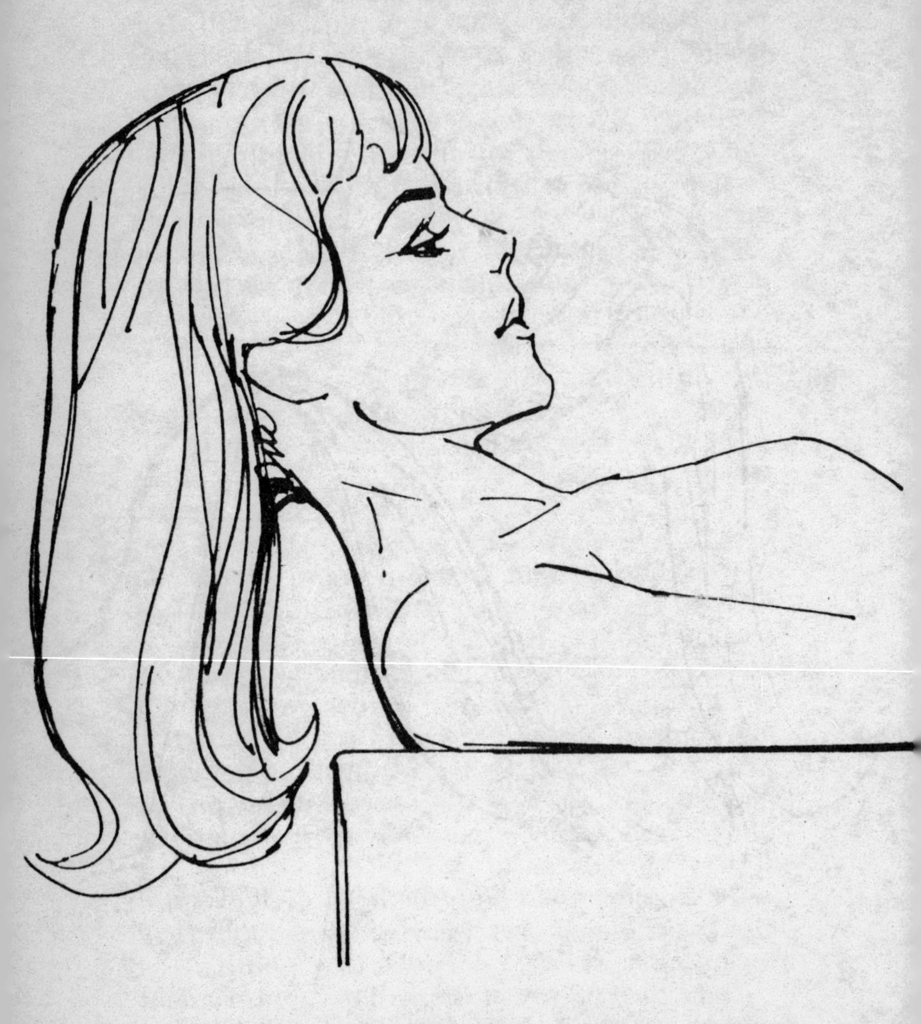

FIG. 25

you raise and lower it to provide resistance. But by lying on the bed, the weight of the head itself, if raised and lowered slowly, provides its own resistance, as your neck muscles will soon testify! Dr. Rossiter stated that the exercise brings into action almost sixty muscles, or thirty pairs. He said, "By development of the neck muscles, the overlying skin will take on a healthier tone, recover its elasticity, and so reduce those folds, creases and deep wrinkles. . . . While you are doing this exercise, if you need proof of muscle activity, put your fingers on your neck just below the chin and jaw. Note the rigid contraction of all the small muscles, and also the contraction of the skin, obliterating loose folds."

Sanford Bennett, "the man who grew young," gave credit for this type of face exercise to Ninon de L'Enclos, the seventeenth century woman who "never grew old." When she was seventy, men still swooned over her. Her face, neck and figure continued to dazzle admirers until she died at the age of ninety-one. She told intimate friends that the exercise developed above was largely responsible for her youthful neck contour.

Sanford Bennett wrote, "In my own case I did not commence these exercises until I was over fifty. You will notice that at that time the loose hanging skin was very marked; while my profile photograph taken at age seventy-two demonstrates my success."

Dr. Rossiter used both the head-neck exercise and the smile-up exercise. He claimed that they took up his "brisket" one inch in a month.

You can produce an immediate improvement in cords of the neck if you do the following:

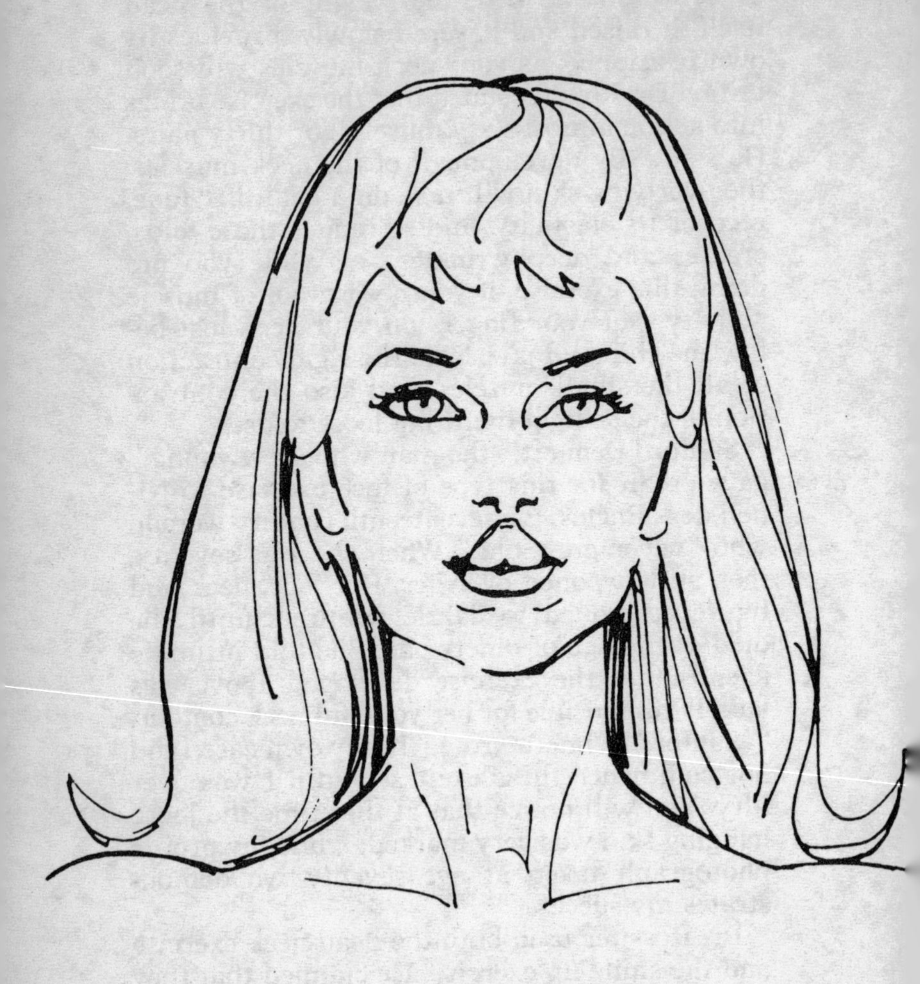

FIG. 26

Drop your shoulders and thrust your collarbone straight forward. Hold this posture as long as possible until gradually it becomes a habit.

Jheri Redding believes that lying on a slant board, tensing and massaging upwards with the fingers held sideways, will greatly diminish the key wrinkles.

Double Chin

Dr. Rossiter suggested sticking out your tongue and trying to touch first the tip of your nose (Fig. 26), and then the end of your chin (Fig. 27). He explained that the "tongue pointing" draws the base of the tongue forward and contracts and pulls all the muscles in the neck.

Vogue magazine recommends this exercise for a firm chin line: "Play at being Eve. Dangle, in your imagination, the reddest, roundest, most succulent apple in the world over your head. Tip your head back, arms down, shoulders relaxed, and reach for that apple with your mouth, imagining that you are biting it hard! Use only the muscles of your throat and neck, and pull, pull, pull toward that apple, then bite it with a vengeance! The apple may be imaginary, the results aren't; a stronger-looking throat; neck visibly longer and more supple; and a good firm tone to the band of muscles under your chin" (Fig. 28).

After presenting this exercise in another book, I received the following letter: "Dear Linda Clark: I approached the apple exercise with healthy skepticism, but some thousands of apples later, I find that my chin and throat are in much

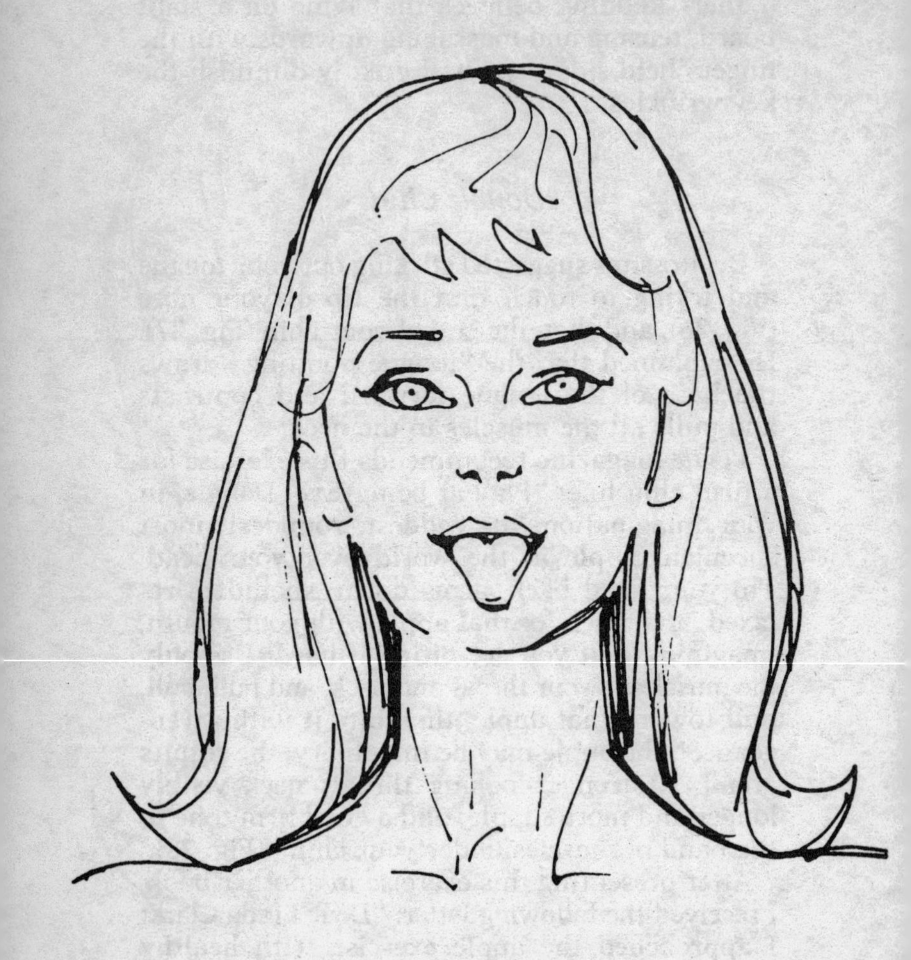

FIG. 27

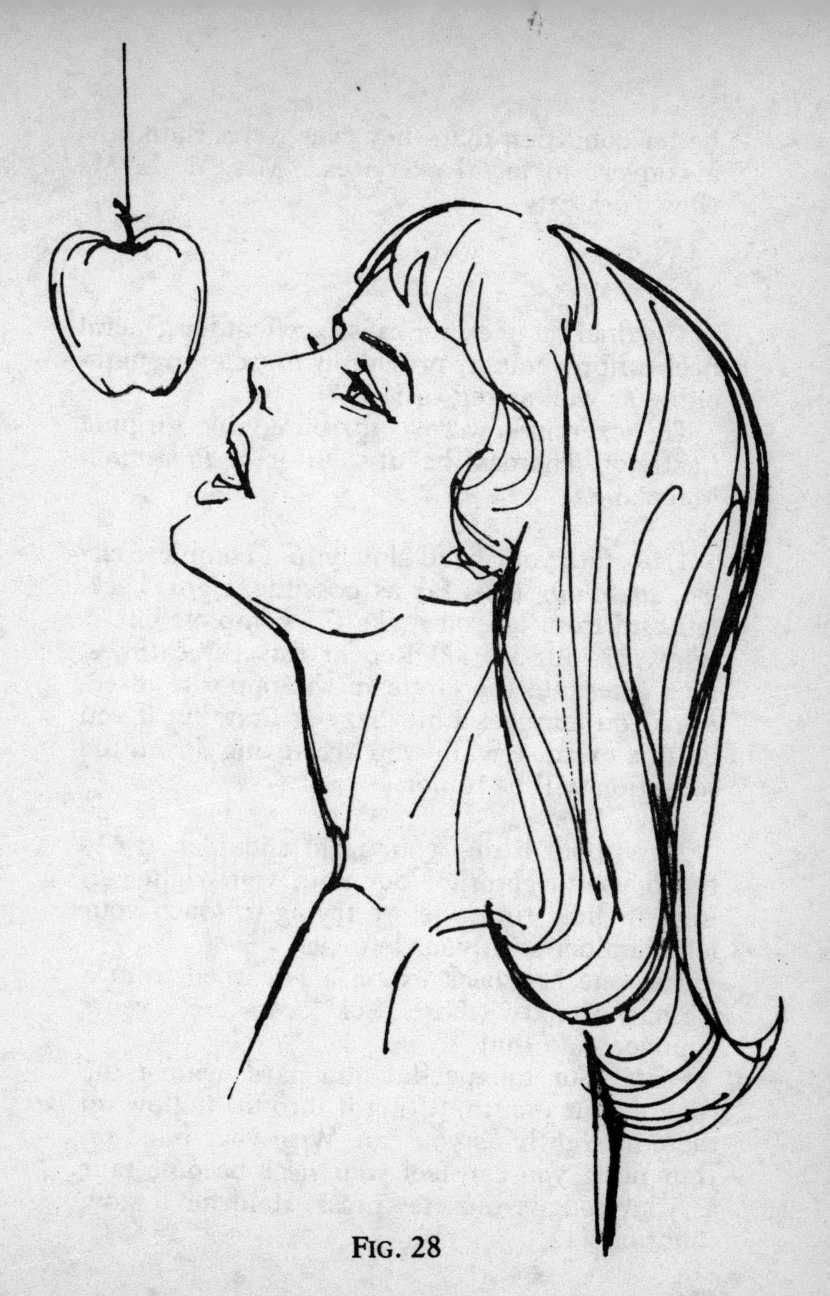

FIG. 28

better condition than they ever were. I am now a convert to facial exercises." Mrs. H. L. M., New York City.

The final set of exercises is excellent for general neck improvement, providing muscle strengthening as well as relaxation.

The exercises were contributed by Virginia Castleton Thomas, beauty editor of *Prevention* Magazine.

1. Rotate your head slowly in a complete circle, *stretching* it as far as possible, right, back, left and front as you make the complete circle. (Figs. 29, 30, 31, 32) Repeat this three times, then alternate the circle in the opposite direction. You may get a bit dizzy at first, but if you do this exercise while you are sitting down, the sensation will be minor.

2. Without lifting your right shoulder, try to touch your right shoulder with your right ear. Repeat three times before trying to touch your left shoulder with your left ear.

And one last neck exercise I learned from a woman of sixty whose neck looks thirty years younger than that.

Press your tongue flat and hard against the roof of your mouth, fitting it into the hollow up there as tightly as you can. With your hand on your neck, you can feel your neck become taut as your tongue muscles press. Hold for a slow count of six.

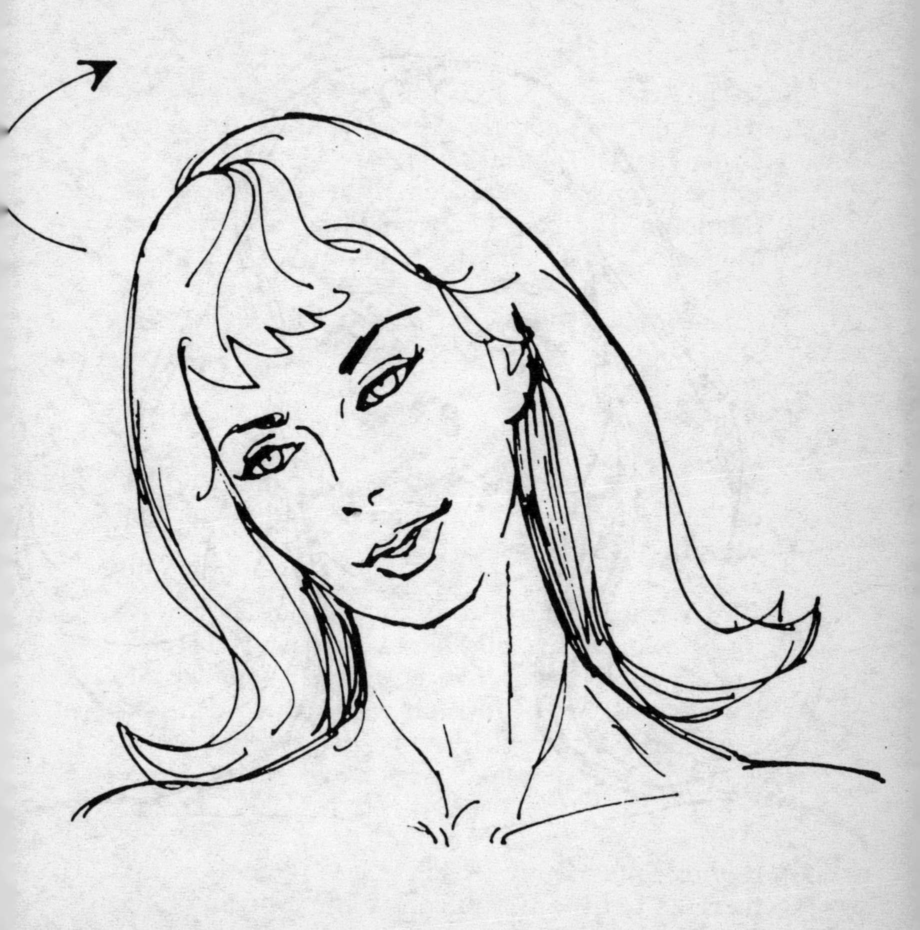

FIG. 29

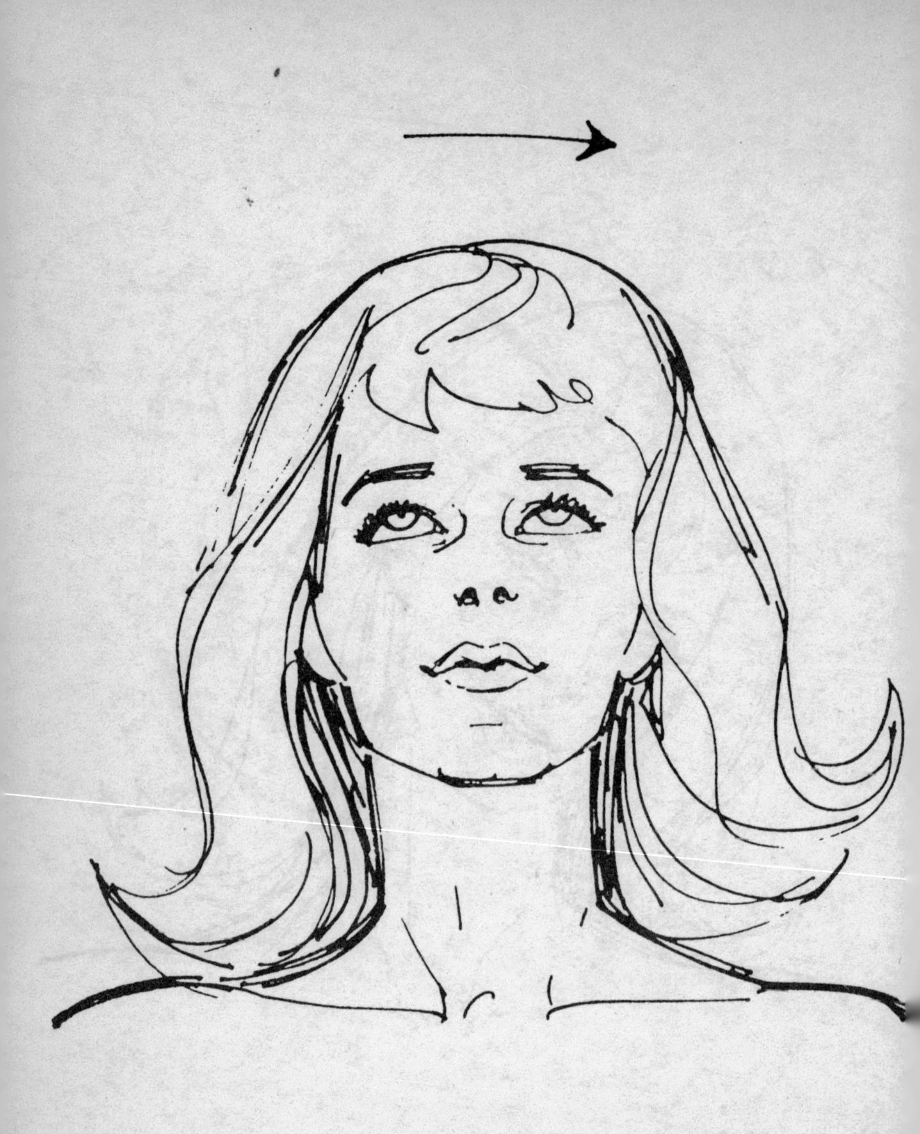

Fig. 30

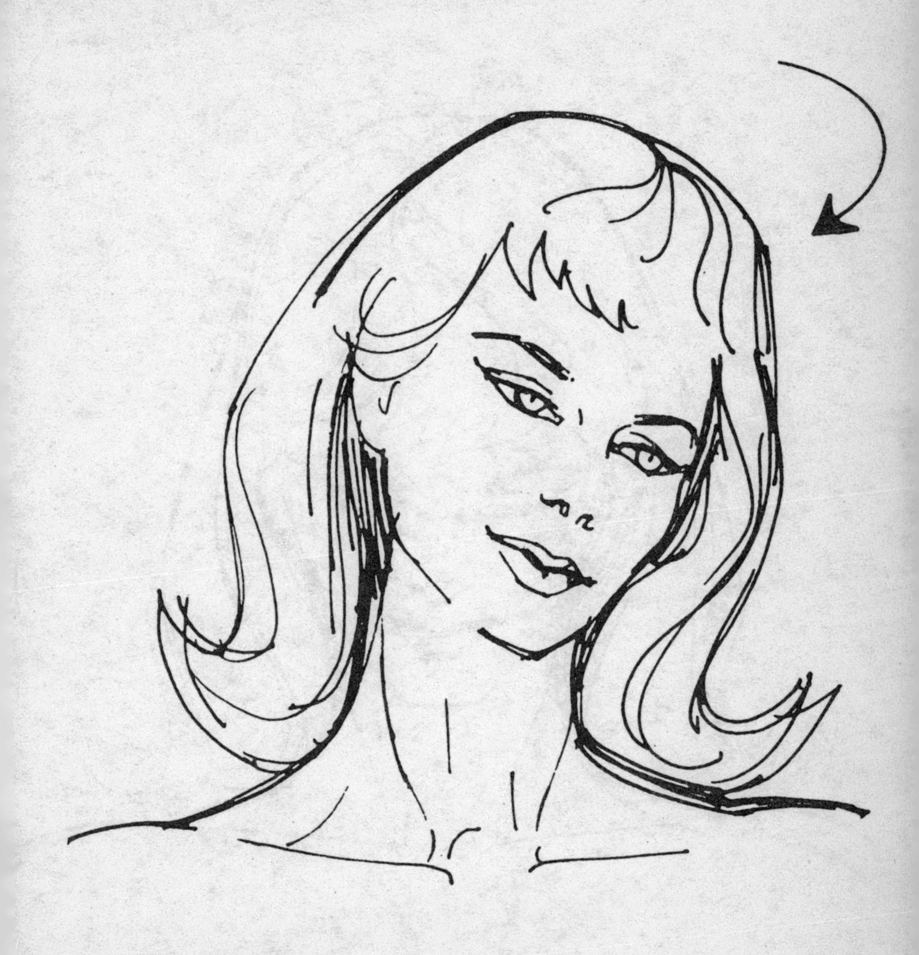

FIG. 31

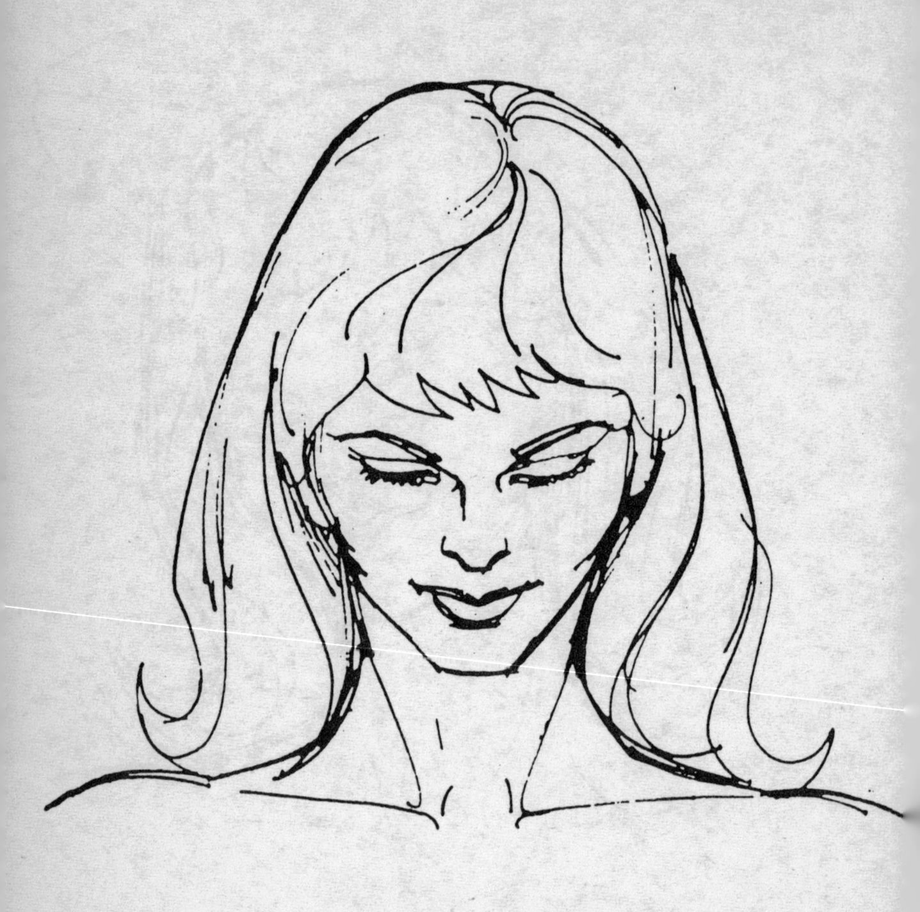

FIG. 32

This concludes your face-exercise regime.

Whichever exercises you choose for your own problems, do them consistently, persistently, automatically. No face exercise that I or anyone else can suggest is sacred! If you find a special problem not covered in this book, make up your own exercise. Now that you understand the principles, you can do it as well as anyone.

Remember always to begin your face exercises and end them with the smile-up exercise, repeating to the point of fatigue.

In time, your family and friends will begin to ask: What are you doing? Do you feel better? Have you been on vacation? They will appear slightly puzzled because they will see a difference they cannot quite pinpoint. Best of all, however, after making a face-exercise program a way of life, you will reach the point where you will no longer dread looking in the mirror. That will be your greatest reward.

Finally, remember that instant face lift when you look at others: Smile!

Index of Illustrations

Text References and Related Books

Bennett, Sanford. *Old Age, Its Cause and Prevention.* New York: Physical Culture Publishing Co., 1912. (Out of print).

Clark, Linda. *Be Slim and Healthy.* New Canaan, Connecticut: Keats Publishing, Inc., 1972.

——. *Help Yourself to Health.* New York: Pyramid Publications. 1972.

——. *Light on Your Health Problems.* New Canaan, Connecticut: Keats Publishing, Inc., 1972.

——. *Stay Younger Longer.* New York: Pyramid Publications. 1968.

——. *Secrets of Health and Beauty.* New York: Pyramid Publications. 1970.

Crane, Jessica. *How to Use Your Hands to Save Your Face.* Hawthorn Books, Inc.

Family Circle magazine. 5.71.

Rossiter, Frederick M. *Face Culture.* New York: Pageant Press, 1956. (Out of print).

San Francisco Chronicle. 3.13.72.

Thomas, Virginia Castleton. *My Secrets of Natural Beauty.* New Canaan, Connecticut: Keats Publishing, Inc. 1972.

Women's Wear Daily. 3.72.

MY FACE IMPROVEMENT DIARY

Date ____

Comment_____________________________________

Date ____

Comment_____________________________________

Date ____

Comment_____________________________________

Date ____

Comment_____________________________________